Essential Oils
in
Spiritual Practice

Working with the Chakras,
Divine Archetypes,
and the Five Great Elements

CANDICE COVINGTON

Healing Arts Press
Rochester, Vermont • Toronto, Canada

Healing Arts Press
One Park Street
Rochester, Vermont 05767
www.HealingArtsPress.com

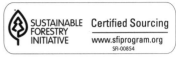

Text stock is SFI certified

Healing Arts Press is a division of Inner Traditions International

Note to the reader: *This book is intended as an informational guide. The remedies, approaches, and techniques described herein are meant to supplement, and not to be a substitute for, professional medical care or treatment. They should not be used to treat a serious ailment without prior consultation with a qualified health care professional.*

Library of Congress Cataloging-in-Publication Data
Names: Covington, Candice, author.
Title: Essential oils in spiritual practice : working with the chakras, divine archetypes, and the five great elements / Candice Covington.
Description: Rochester, Vermont : Healing Arts Press, 2017. | Includes bibliographical references and index.
Identifiers: LCCN 2017026073 (print) | LCCN 2017014153 (e-book) | ISBN 9781620553053 (pbk.) | ISBN 9781620553060 (e-book)
Subjects: LCSH: Essences and essential oils—Miscellanea. | Tattvas (Sankhya)—Miscellanea. | Chakras. | Energy medicine.
Classification: LCC BF1442.E77 (print) | LCC BF1442.E77 C68 2017 (e-book) | DDC 133/.2—dc23
LC record available at https://lccn.loc.gov/2017014153

Printed and bound in the United States by Lake Book Manufacturing, Inc. The text stock is SFI certified. The Sustainable Forestry Initiative® program promotes sustainable forest management.

10 9 8 7 6 5 4 3 2 1

Text design and layout by Virginia Scott Bowman
This book was typeset in Garamond Premier Pro and Gill Sans with Playfair and Cronos Pro used as display typefaces
Illustrations by Maeve Callahan

To send correspondence to the author of this book, mail a first-class letter to the author c/o Inner Traditions • Bear & Company, One Park Street, Rochester, VT 05767, and we will forward the communication, or contact the author directly at **www.divinearchetypes.org**.

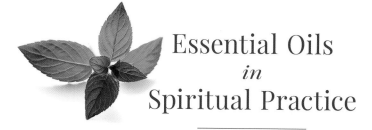

Essential Oils
in
Spiritual Practice

"Before formal analytic analysis, before formal scientific methods, people asked questions about reality and focused on observations of the world and on subjective experience. Theories of outer and inner reality were a part of every culture and every spiritual tradition. From the perspective of contemporary Western science, many of these systems are hard to understand and integrate with our worldview. In particular, systems that use and incorporate subjective experience may seem intuitively powerful, yet they remain difficult to integrate into our sense of reality and are therefore difficult to believe. Candice Covington does a brilliant job of explaining Vedic understanding and the five elements and integrating this worldview with contemporary archetypal psychology and contemporary scientific thinking. This is a good and powerful read. Challenge yourself and enjoy."

CHRISTINE G. GLENN, PSY.D.,
CLINICAL PSYCHOLOGIST IN PORTLAND, OREGON

"An exceptionally talented woman, whose words are as beautiful as the aromas she creates, Candice Covington has now created a must-have book for anyone interested in spirituality, ayurveda, and the subtle use of essential oils. Profound and engaging, this book is a worthy and important addition to any aromatic library."

SHELLIE ENTEEN, R.A., L.M.B.T., WRITER,
AROMATHERAPIST, AND WORKSHOP TEACHER

"I was so excited to read this book! Weaving wisdom traditions with contemporary science, depth psychology, and personal dreams, Candice offers a bold vision and a wealth of practical applications for working with essential oils and vibrational remedies. In her exploration of Lilith and Snake as potently creative shadow archetypes, she does not shy away from naming the importance of consciously embracing the primordial depths to facilitate lasting change. If you want to understand how transformation and deep healing actually work, this book is a must-read!"

ANDREA MATHIESON, CREATOR OF
THE RAVEN ESSENCE PROJECT AND EARTHSONG MYSTERIES

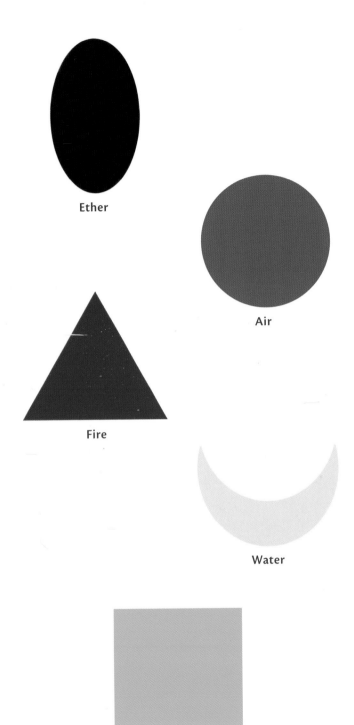

The five elemental yantras; sacred geometry of the tattvas

To the vast wonders above, below,
and all spaces in between

Contents

PART 3

Healing Practices

❧

Foreword

It is well established that who we *really* are is not only the physical molecules that make up our body but also the energy that suffuses our being and expresses itself through our thoughts and feelings. Ultimately, we are the awareness of our physical sensations and thoughts. Studies in neuroscience have shown that we can influence our cells (and thus our physical body) by applying electromagnetic fields to the body and that our own body maintains subtle energy fields that can be influenced by our thoughts and intentions. An imbalance in any layer of our existence can cause disruption in the entire system. In other words, an imbalance in the subtle energy body can cause both emotional turbulence and physical illness. In my practice as a medical doctor, I have often come across situations where the "solution" did not lie at the level of biomolecules or matter. Before developing an understanding of ourselves as fields of energy and awareness, I had nothing to offer patients to further their healing if medications or medical procedures didn't work. In this book the author offers an approach to healing that addresses the subtle layer of who we are: a field of energy, one that can be influenced by the vibrational and energetic qualities of nature. She gives us the information and tools to address the root cause of our imbalances and maximize our healing abilities.

In the typical Western medical model we use a very Newtonian,

mechanistic viewpoint of who we are, which is only an approxima-
tion of reality, and ultimately an illusion. This approach to healing
does not give us access to the myriad healing modalities that influence
the subtler nature of who we are. This is why I see so many patients
who have been to doctor after doctor only to become more confused,
and often more sick, in the end. A new paradigm of healing is emerg-
ing in which we can address our underlying energy fields, below our
physical/cellular domain. As we shift from a material, Newtonian paradigm toward a more holistic viewpoint, we gain access to powerful
forms of energetic healing.

In this book a gifted healer describes an ancient method of energy
healing in a way that anyone can understand. She beautifully lays out
the theory and rationale behind the use of essential oils, tattvas, and
divine archetypes. This method does not directly address our physical
body, as Western medicine does, but instead engages our subtle energy
body. Healers have used this type of energy healing for millennia to
remove obstructions that have gotten in the way of us experiencing
our true, balanced nature. These time-tested methods provide us with
a system of subtle energy medicine that can encourage deep healing
and vibrant well-being.

When I first met Candice, I was familiar with the theories of
our underlying nature of vibration and energy, but through her work
with essential oils and tattvas, I was able to experience firsthand the
power of our internal energies. Since experiencing this healing modal-
ity myself, I have begun offering it to my own patients, and I can see
the transformation that happens when we begin to affect the deepest
layers of who we are.

With extensive research, self-study, and personal experience, a
gifted and knowledgeable alchemist gives readers a practical guide
toward applying energetic healing through essential oils, tattvas, and
divine archetypes to foster their own healing. If you are feeling stuck

in your healing process, I encourage you to use this guide as a way to move toward your natural state of wholeness, health, and happiness.

Sheila Patel, M.D.
Medical Director, Chopra Center for Wellbeing
Carlsbad, California

Sheila Patel is a board-certified family physician who practiced full-spectrum family medicine—from prenatal care and deliveries to ER coverage and primary care for all ages—for more than a decade. At the Chopra Center, Dr. Patel offers integrative medical consultations that combine the best in conventional medicine with the wisdom of ayurveda. Dr. Patel also serves as the clinical director for the Chopra Center's research team. She enjoys the opportunity to bring light to the mechanisms of action of mind-body practices, giving them scientific validation. She is a volunteer faculty member at the University of California, San Diego (UCSD) School of Medicine and has served as a guest lecturer at several integrative medical conferences as well as at Bastyr University in San Diego.

Acknowledgments

To all of my friends and loved ones who held my hand and encouraged me along the way, deep thanks. I would like to give special thanks to Nancy Thurston, who opened up condo 18 as a hallowed creative space and was endlessly encouraging and such a dear friend; to Ra., who spent countless hours talking theory with me as I fleshed out ideas, and for being a true friend through and through; to Denise P. for her sweet support and love; to Charles Daniels for getting me started and Charlie Shapiro for all his help and keen insight; to Dr. Glenn for sharing her wisdom and kindness; to the Cook family for opening their hearts and homes to me, in particular my dear Curtis; to my Chopra family, especially Shey Shey, Moni j., and Bunny Kelie, for creating a fertile, supportive space for me to grow, learn, and love in; to Dr. Sheila Patel for writing such a beautiful foreword and for carving out a niche for me to bring my theories to life and making it possible for me to practice them in such a rarefied place; and to Jamaica and Nancy, the sweetest, most patient editors on earth, who helped me more than I can say.

PART 1

Theory

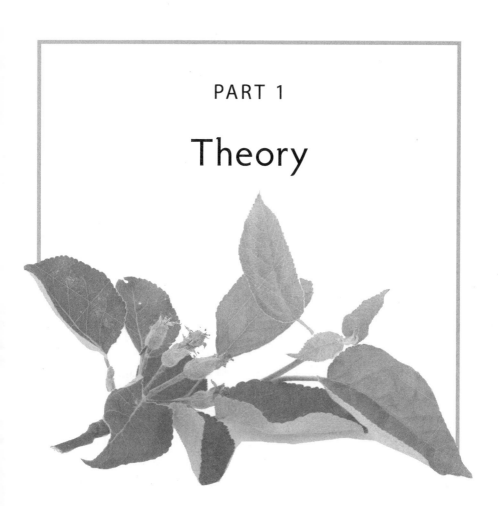

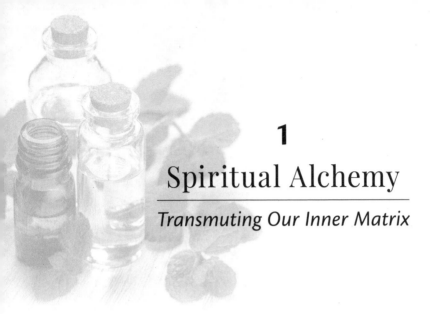

1

Spiritual Alchemy

Transmuting Our Inner Matrix

Alchemy can be defined as any magical power or process of transmuting a common substance, usually of little value, into a substance of great value.[1] Early alchemists are best remembered for their attempts to transmute lead into gold. Over the centuries, the concept of alchemy has grown from its foundation in metallurgy to encompass psychological and spiritual transmutation. Dr. Carl Jung's work, for example, focused on the alchemical transmutation of shadow into light, or the transformation of leaden aspects of the self into enlightened, golden aspects of the self. And modern spiritual traditions invoke the power of alchemy in the transmutation of the self from a singular inward-turning consciousness to one that is awakened, dynamic, and open to the subtle energies around us.

Traditions of energy healing—that is, activating, supporting, or unblocking the body's own subtle energy fields to facilitate healing and well-being—can be seen as a form of spiritual alchemy. In restoring a balanced flow of energy through the body, energy healing brings us back into alignment with universal energies, or the Source from which all form and energy emanate. Thus aligned, our consciousness opens; our inner matrix meshes with the world around us, and we are drawn to the path toward our highest self.

If we intend to undertake the spiritual alchemy of our own inner matrix, we must begin by exploring what that matrix is made of. That conversation begins with the concept of vibration.

The Vibrational Universe

Every manifestation of matter in the universe—human, animal, or inanimate object, from atoms to organisms to galaxies—vibrates according to its own unique signature, or vibrational pattern. We are all manifestations of vibration, a form of energy, and so we are all at a foundational level beings of energy. Deepak Chopra explains this beautifully.

> So the physical world, the world of objects and matter, is made up of nothing but information contained in energy vibrating at different frequencies. The reason we don't see the world as a huge web of energy is that it is vibrating far too fast. Our senses, because they function so slowly, are able to register only chunks of this energy and activity, and these clusters of information become "the chair," "my body," "water," and every other physical object in the visible universe.[2]

Knowing that matter is made up of energy vibrating at different frequencies, it is fascinating to consider our own vibrational signature as human beings. Researcher Warren J. Hamerman notes that the organic matter that forms human beings generates a frequency that can be represented by sound at approximately forty-two octaves above middle C (the note near the center of the piano keyboard), or roughly 570 trillion Hz. Because Hz (the Hertz scale) measures vibrations per second, what we're saying is that human beings vibrate 570 trillion times a second, a number that exceeds the imagination and indicates incredible and wonderful hidden potential.[3]

That fantastically huge number becomes even harder to comprehend when we point out that the frequency of the human being is immensely diverse. Each atom, cell, structure, and organ of the body vibrates according to its own unique pattern. The human being holds a universe within, filled with overlapping frequencies, and the result is a symphony of cosmic proportions.

Buddha proclaimed long ago that a human being comes in and out of solidity sixty times in the course of one second. Whether Buddha or Hamerman is correct, the point is simple and astounding: We vibrate—we come in and out of solidity—constantly, continuously, and at a rate so fast it's hard to imagine. That gives us a lot of wiggle room for rearranging ourselves into patterns that serve our highest being.

Vibrational Healing

Physics shows us that vibrations can affect one another across space and time in an interplay of frequency (the rate of vibration) and amplitude (the strength of vibration). The principle of *resonance* describes the way in which one vibration can reinforce another: when one vibration induces vibration in another object—the air in a trombone, a seashell, or a drum, for example—at its natural frequency, that object vibrates with greater amplitude. In other words, resonance builds a vibration that is louder, more stable, or more powerful.

Because we are vibrational beings in a constant state of flux, a significant key to our well-being and growth is reinforcement of our desired energetic patterns. We must learn to recognize inharmonic patterns in ourselves, identify vibrational tools with a strong, stable, resonant frequency, and use those tools to transmute the inharmonic energy into a beneficial form. In other words, we can purposefully introduce outside vibrational energies to positively influence, through the power of resonance, our own natural signature, or vibrational pattern.

The natural world, with its vast and wondrous array of forms and energies, offers us a treasure trove of vibrational tools that we can use as antidotes for negative energetic patterns and supports for the cultivation of positive qualities. The vibration of each plant, mineral, or stone can be understood as an energy pattern with a specific and unique structure, or signature. When these energetic signatures resonate with our natural vibrational patterns, we can use them to precisely fine-tune our own energetic bodies.

Jungian analyst E. C. Whitmont tells us, "Every pattern of adaptation, outer and inner, is maintained in essentially the same unaltered form and anxiously defended against change until an equally strong or stronger impulse is able to displace it."[4] In other words, when our energetic patterns—our vibrations—encounter a purer, stronger pattern, the new pattern serves as a template for reformatting the old pattern. The vibrational signatures of plants, minerals, metals, and gems offer the architecture of a stable foundation onto which we can consciously craft our inner matrix and transform our outer reality. In other words, they are vibrational tools for spiritual alchemy.

Even more fascinating is the idea that energy never dissipates; it simply changes form. The visionary biochemist and philosopher Rupert Sheldrake reminds us, "For example, if a bunch of flowers are thrown into a furnace and reduced to ashes, the total amount of matter and energy remains the same, but the form of the flowers simply disappears."[5] This is important to understand when we are doing personal work. We are not getting rid of something; we are changing the form of our own personal *aggregates*—the energy, matter, and patterns that, taken all together, make us *us*. This is such a liberating understanding: Our woundings, shortcomings, and negative behavioral patterns are not *us*! They are, for visualization purposes, vibrational imprints pressed into the clay of our being, and we are capable of skillfully transmuting *their very energy* into its beneficial form.

My favorite definition of the term *aggregates* is "the components of the psycho-physical personality, on the basis of which beings commonly impute the false notion of self."[6] This is a rich concept to sit with. So much of what we feel guilt about or struggle with is a false notion of self. The judicious use of vibrational tools can act as an antidote to the wounds surrounding our false notion of self, freeing us from the web of illusion and allowing us to move into the flow of our life purpose without restraint.

Archetypal Energies and Our Collective Reality

Carl Jung is perhaps the best-known proponent of the idea of a collective reality, which he described as the *collective unconscious,* or an inherited set of thoughtforms common to all humans and feeding the unconscious from a universal wellspring of patterns. In other words, the energetic patterns arising from Source (or God, or the universe, or whatever font of creation you might choose to believe in) imbue each of us with certain preset ways of perceiving and understanding reality. As Jung explains:

> It means that there are present in every psyche forms which are unconscious but nonetheless active—living dispositions, ideas in the Platonic sense, that preform and continually influence our thoughts and feelings and actions.[7]

In many Eastern creation stories, from Vedanta to Buddhism, the world is said to have begun as an emanation of form out of the emptiness of pure potential. From this perspective, which echoes Jung's, everything in creation is a specific pattern that has risen out of the universal ether and collated into a recognizable form.

Philosopher Rupert Sheldrake has proposed a similar theory whereby morphogenesis (the process by which organisms and structures take form) is guided by *morphic fields,* or energetic organizational patterns that determine the development of forms. Sheldrake describes the array of morphic fields as a universal database for both organic (living) and abstract (mental) forms. He notes:

The approach I am putting forward is very similar to Jung's idea of the collective unconscious. The main difference is that Jung's idea was applied primarily to human experience and human collective memory. What I am suggesting is that a very similar principle operates through the entire universe, not just human beings.[8]

Whether you call them the *collective unconscious* or *morphic fields,* the complex thoughtforms that underlie our perception of reality can be understood as organizers of ideas that ultimately lead to forms (the structures we apprehend) and behaviors (the ways in which forms interact). An *archetype* can be thought of as a model that embodies an aspect of the collective unconscious. It is a particular idea or pattern arising from our collective unconscious or universal Source and giving shape to forms and behaviors.

As an example, let's consider the archetype of the moon and its eternal cycle of transmutation. The "dark moon" period is the approximately three-day stretch during which the moon is invisible to the human eye, because it rises and sets with the sun. From this "death" comes the new moon.

THE ARCHETYPE OF THE MOON: TRANSMUTATION

The transmutation of the moon can be seen as an archetype for transmutation of the self, or spiritual alchemy. You can see this archetype manifesting with similar symbolism in the mythology of many cultures. (This is a fascinating demonstration of the fact that archetypes are universal concepts—their patterning appears over and over, in manifold forms resonating with similar energy.)

In her cycle from dark moon to full moon and back again, the moon undergoes a rite of passage every month: she grows to fulfillment (full moon), is unable to hold that position, falls into decay, and finally lies dormant as if dead for three days (dark moon), to be born again in exquisite light. The example the moon sets in this context is powerfully instructive. As Jungian analyst Jules Cashford notes:

> This is to say that, at the deepest level, we could infer that modes of feeling, thinking and being experience themselves as perpetually in movement, growing and diminishing and reforming to a rhythm of their own. Arising from invisible depths, they take on a shape and a character, growing to their most complete manifestation, after which, their purpose done, they start to dwindle, their conviction fades, and (if we would let them) they dissolve back into a deeper stratum of the psyche where they can be re-absorbed, refreshed, and reborn in new form, one more in accord with what has been learned through this latest expression of themselves.[9]

The idea that knowledge or enlightenment is an energy that grows and evolves in cycles is often represented by Snake, one of the animal totems associated with the moon. Again, we turn to Cashford.

> Serpents, sloughing their skin as the Moon its shadow, are believed to be continually reborn like the Moon and so to share in the Moon's powers of renewal. Like the Dark Moon they vanish, leaving their old skin behind in winter and hibernating until spring when they return new-born. In this way they are epiphanies of the self-consuming and self-renewing powers of life, the mystery of an energy beyond the forms of time. . . . If there were any further doubt about the Moon/serpent correlation, Aristotle states as a fact in his *History of Animals* that serpents have as many ribs as there are days in the lunar month (200 is apparently a closer estimate).[10]

Snake's symbolization of knowledge moving into higher levels of understanding can be seen in its embodiment in kundalini ("coiled one"), a primal energy that winds its way up through our chakras, starting in the first (muladhara) chakra, related to base survival issues, up through the seventh (sahasrara) chakra, which holds the energy of enlightenment. Kundalini, or the snake, spiraling her way upward is the embodiment of evolution through cycles of growth, death, and rebirth. This idea—that authentic growth requires multiple life-death-rebirths so that we can acquire the wisdom we need to progress—is expressed in almost every culture on Earth.

Hebraic-Christian texts express this truth with the story of Jonah, who spent three days in the belly of a whale, and Jesus, who lay dead for three days in the heart of the earth before his resurrection. "For as Jonah was three days and three nights in the whale's belly; so shall the Son of man be three days and three nights in the heart of the earth" (Matthew 12:40).

The Sumerian culture has a similar myth, as does Egypt and East India.

It was for three days and three nights that the Sumerian Moon goddess, Inanna, hung dead as a corpse upon a hook in the Great Below until, revived by the water and food of life, she ascended back into the Great Above. It was for three nights that the Left Eye of Horus was torn into pieces and thrown into outer darkness, when Thoth reassembled it, piecing it together until it was whole. . . . In Vedic India, the souls who died into the old Moon were reincarnated three nights later in the returning crescent, falling into the wombs of their new mothers as *Soma*-rain.[11]

These myths allude to the three-day period of the dark moon, when the moon rises and sets with the sun and so is hidden from human sight. The new moon that rises into the sky as a sliver crescent holds the energy of rebirth, the promise of spring, the power of new beginnings birthed from the primordial womb of the dark moon phase.

However, the promise of a new beginning—of death, rebirth, and growth—can feel frightening if the change is an uninvited one. In the tarot, this concept is taught as the Tower, or the idea that once a powerful citadel offering security becomes a limiting prison, the walls must come down to allow new life in. As we all know, when the wheel of life moves forward, there is no stopping it. Anyone who has lost a relationship, employment, a friendship, or simply an aspect of self that needed to be shed can relate to this energy.

The archetype of the moon addresses not only how to move into a new cycle of growth, ready or not, but how to gain the overarching perspective that allows us to see that the cycle of loss leads to new gain. This allows us to experience personal rebirth without fear, resentment, or anger and to see the truth of the situation. It is vital to acknowledge that the dark moon phase is about composting. If we are willing to dig deep into the compost of the cycle that came before, or the dark womb's "three days of darkness," we will have all that we need to flourish in the new moon phase.

This is where the combination of focused intent, surrender to the natural rhythms of life, and the use of essential oils and other vibrational tools can be useful, for they allow us access to the very strata of our being. These tools work on the deeper levels of self to facilitate shifts in our energetic body, which will in turn affect the conscious self, allowing more of our essence self to emerge. Ariel Spilsbury, author of *The Mayan Oracle,* defines *essence self* as "the eternal higher self or true self, the 'I Am' presence that is unlimited by ego, mind, concepts, or definitions."[12] The more we allow our self to be in process and authentically shed old skins of conditioned ways of being, the closer we come to finding our true face.

This begs the question, "What did your face look like before your parents were born?" This Zen koan invites us to recognize the empty nature of reality by looking beyond the particulars of our cultural and psychological understanding of self, body, and mind. It is truly a new moon question! Who are you, when you are not defined by outside factors?

I was shown a fledgling learning to fly,
Its first efforts were very feeble,
but as it used its wings more and more,
they became stronger
until it found the freedom of flight
and was able to soar to great heights
and fly great distances without any effort.
I heard the words:
"Faith comes with practice.
Live by faith until it becomes rocklike and
*   unshakable*
and find the true freedom of the spirit."[13]

We, like the fledgling, are strengthening our new wings in the new moon phase of this cycle. Until we can take flight, we must live by faith that the undertakings in this cycle will flourish.

One of the difficulties of a recent rebirth from the amniotic fluid of the dark moon—the heart of any transmutative effort—is that often we need a gentle spark to ignite the journey (similar to the way that a newborn baby often needs gentle stimulation to ensure that its breathing reflexes kick in). Birthing the self can be a traumatic, exhausting experience, leaving us drained. This is where having access to the energetic blueprint of a specific archetypal energy can help us move into our new way of being.

USING ARCHETYPAL ENERGY

In a quest for spiritual alchemy, we seek transmutation of the self— that is, we aim to transform and elevate our inner matrix to a place of greater communion with the energies that surround us, from people and animals to the Earth and the environment to the very universe itself. Knowing that the moon manifests the archetypal energy for transmutation, we can turn to it in meditation, reflection, artistic expression, ritual, and other practices to evoke its energy in ourselves.

The moon becomes that spark we need to motivate us to stay steadfast on the journey toward our highest self.

The archetypal energy of transmutation can also be seen in other forms, like ether, one of the five tattvas (see chapter 3), and betel leaf essential oil, a powerful vibrational tool (see chapter 6). These forms express the archetypal energy of transmutation strongly and, like the moon, can be used as tools to awaken that energy in ourselves.

Every form in the world holds the energy of archetypes, including plants, minerals, and human beings. With conscious intention, we can use an archetype to access a facet of the collective unconscious, or Source, and awaken that energy inside us. But because we are all part of that collective unconscious, or Source, we are not attempting to incorporate an aspect outside of ourselves but rather to awaken to an existing aspect that lies dormant within us. That archetypal energy of transmutation is already part of us; we have only to access it, ignite it, and set it free.

> *A new moon teaches gradualness*
> *and deliberation and how one gives birth*
> *to oneself slowly. Patience with small details*
> *makes perfect a large work, like the universe.*
>
> RUMI

The Bridge

Energy runs both ways across the bridge from the collective unconscious to self—that is, archetypes shape us, but we also shape archetypes. In elevating our inner matrix with spiritual practice, we also elevate the development of humankind and the universe at large.

Our culture generally adheres to the idea of a fixed inherent nature—that our inner self remains true and unchangeable throughout our life, and we simply must learn to work with what we have been born with, and that, likewise, the world around us is built from set forms and behaviors. In other words, as the popular expression goes, "a leopard cannot change its spots."

This idea of a fixed existence does not allow for the interplay of physical and psychological energies in reshaping reality. However, we are going to explore methods that allow us to rearrange not only our interior vibrational fields but also the archetypal energetic fields that create our collective reality.

Jung remarkably foretold such a concept.

Sooner or later nuclear physics and the psychology of the unconscious will draw closely together as both of them, independently of one another and from opposite directions, push forward into transcendental territory, the one with the concept of the atom, the other with that of the archetype.

The analogy with physics is not a digression since the symbolical schema itself represents the descent into matter and requires the identity of the outside with the inside. Psyche cannot be totally different from matter, for how otherwise could it move matter? And matter cannot be alien to psyche, for how else could matter produce psyche? Psyche and matter exist in one and the same world, and each partakes of the other, otherwise any reciprocal action would be impossible. If research could only advance far enough, therefore, we should arrive at an ultimate agreement between physical and psychological concepts. Our present attempts may be bold, but I believe they are on the right lines. Mathematics, for instance, has more than once proved that its purely logical constructions which transcend all experience subsequently coincided with the behavior of things. This, like the events I call synchronistic, points to a profound harmony between all forms of existence.[14]

This agreement between physical and psychological concepts is the juncture at which vibrational remedies come into play as powerful healing tools for well-being and spiritual alchemy. When we feel stuck in an inharmonic pattern—a behavior or form that does not serve our highest self—no matter how deeply embedded or "you" an issue/pattern may feel, it is possible for a leopard to change its spots. A significant key to human growth is identifying patterns and then finding the means to heal the inharmonic ones, transmuting the inharmonic energy into a beneficial form. With vibrational tools we can access not only our own personal disharmonies but also those of the world at large, taking advantage of the bridge between the collective unconscious and our own energetic cord to ignite a powerful alchemy of enlightenment.

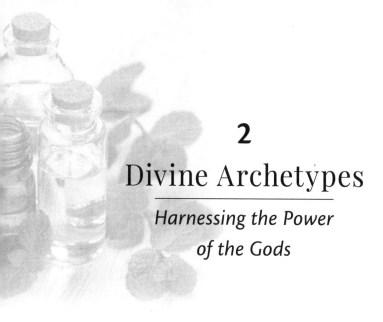

2

Divine Archetypes

Harnessing the Power of the Gods

Knowing that archetypes shape the manifestation of form and behavior, we can look to archetypal manifestations as models of forms and/or behaviors that we wish to embody ourselves. This brings us to the idea of *divine* archetypes: archetypes embodied by gods and goddesses from around the world. These divinities arose in our mythologies by virtue of archetypal energies; they manifest universal patterns of form and behavior arising from the collective unconscious in a manner that we, as natural storytellers, can access and understand. This is not to demean or undermine the power of the religions from which these gods and goddesses hail. Rather, understanding gods and goddesses as archetypes lends credibility to their power and sacredness. They are the epitome of Source, God, Mother Goddess, the universe—of creation and the power that drives it. Seeing them as archetypes simply recognizes their divine origin.

Static information is useless, so in this chapter we will explore how to apply the information offered by these divine energy complexes on a practical level. We will review how to invoke divine archetypal energy, what specific patterns can do for you, and basic concepts dealing with essential oils within this context.

Divine Archetypes in
Spiritual Practice

Divine archetypes are particularly helpful in spiritual practice because they are easy to access and understand. A god (or goddess) generally has an ample mythology built up around him, and therefore we can readily grasp the qualities, traits, and energies he represents. Compared to an unshaped, unmanifest aspect of the collective unconscious that we might have trouble invoking, we can easily call upon a god(dess) to help us, and we can use that divine archetype as an energetic blueprint to shape our own energetic body, allowing a change in behavior, emotions, or mental state. A divine archetype offers a tried-and-true template refined over time to achieve goals such as personal betterment, ease of pain, and making the world a better place. The key is to identify which divine archetype most supports our goals.

Repatterning:
Mobilizing Archetypal Energies

An established divine archetype emanates the tremendous energy contained within its morphic field. When we invoke such an archetypal energy pattern, we call up a very strong, clear blueprint that we can use as a template to shape our energetic self.

Repatterning is a technique taught in Tibetan schools of Buddhism in which advanced students will engage in visualizations of a particular deity that they wish not simply to emulate but to actually become, merging their personal energetic field with that of the deity before melting into emptiness. This repatterning concept offers the possibility of rapid growth. Author John Powers, in his textbook on Tibetan Buddhism, writes, "The buddha's wisdom consciousness,* motivated by

---

Wisdom consciousness is the totality of an individual psychological process, including both the consciousness and unconscious in a luminous state.

compassion, is a projection of one's own mind and serves as a template for one's development."[1]

Here again we are reminded: We are not learning a principle outside of self but rather awaking to an aspect within self. The deity we invoke is an archetype we can use as a template to shape our energetic body and stimulate a positive shift.

Invoking a divine archetype for repatterning requires direct, active engagement with the energy you wish to embody. It is analogous to learning how to ride a bike. You could ask individuals who ride bikes about their techniques and methodology and read the manual that comes with your bike to discover the nuts and bolts of a bike's construction. In doing this, you will gain a general understanding of what you are working with and some proven strategies for riding a bike. So it is true to say that you have a mental understanding of how to ride a bike and what a bike is. But anyone who ever learned how to ride a bike knows that reading about it is a far cry from mastering it. Direct engagement with the bike is required—you have to climb into the saddle and push off before you can master the skill. The same principle of total engagement holds true for working with archetypes—you must invoke an archetype to learn to use its energy.

Archetypal Energies: Alternative Views

The Buddhists are quick to remind us that when we invoke archetypal energies, we are awakening and developing dormant aspects of self, rather than asking outside energies to enter us. On the other hand, the followers of Voodoo, or Vodun, view archetypal patterns as external energetic forms that they call Loa. In one healing Vodun ritual, the Loa are called in from the outside to take possession of an individual, and the host is healed by the presence of the spirit. Possession by a Loa is considered a positive and dynamic means of growth and healing.

The followers of Vodun believe that each person has a soul

composed of two parts: a *gros bon ange*, "big guardian angel," and a *ti bon ange*, "little guardian angel." When a Loa is called in the "little guardian angel" leaves the body and the Loa takes its place. Often this is brought about by dancing led by the *houngan* (male Vodun priest) and/or *mambo* (female Vodun priest). The dancing will typically build in intensity until one of the dancers becomes possessed by a Loa and falls. The possessed dancer will behave as the Loa and is treated with respect and ceremony by the others present.

The Loa possession ceremony is considered "white" magic, which is used to bring good fortune and healing. We can easily see the correlation between the "little guardian angel" and the "conscious self" and how the Vodun system "summons" the archetypal energy (the Loa) through ritual, completely displacing the conscious mind for a while. Individuals who have hosted the Loa often report that they have no recollection of their experience, but the energy of the Loa facilitated a change in them or for them.

Using Essential Oils to Invoke Divine Archetypes

In both my personal and professional experience I have found essential oils to be catalysts for profound change. Through their energetic properties they play a significant role in addressing what Jung terms *psychic inertia,* where a conscious mental shift alone is not enough to rid us of deeper, unwanted psychological influences. Essential oils help us achieve the shift in our energetic body that is required for bringing about a deeper, lasting change.

This, of course, assumes that we have already identified the change we desire. However, it is often the case that although we wish to make a change, we do not necessarily know what that change might be or how to go about making it. In such cases, it is possible to use essential oils to identify the archetypal energy that would best serve us. We can simply set our intention to choose an essential oil that resonates with the archetypal energy we most need and then allow the vibrational energy of the oils to guide our choice; see chapter 11 for more details.

When we identify a divine archetype we wish to embody, we can use a corresponding essential oil to repattern our own energies to bring us into alignment with the archetype, thus awakening the dormant aspect of self that we wish to develop. This helps us escape our psychic inertia and can propel us forward on the path to our desired transformation.

Clearing the Slate: Purification

It is possible to engage with the energetic blueprint of a divine archetype and achieve a spontaneous understanding and embodiment. However, the more refined and clear your own energetic body is, the more sensitively it can respond. That is why most traditional practices include intensive preliminary steps to purify and cleanse any negative/obscuring energetic patterns in the beginning of the process of growth.

Essential oils and other vibrational tools can dynamically support the overall purification process. Hemlock spruce, tulsi (holy basil), and white birch are especially helpful in the purification process; see chapter 6 for details.

Multiplicities of Form

Archetypal energy can take on different patterns as it rises up from your depths to communicate with you. It can be fascinating to see what emanation or form it will take and how each aspect expresses the same message. For example, the Dark Goddess archetype can manifest in goddess form but also as a black oval, the dark moon, or a snake; all tell the same story, and in fact the unconscious sees all as the same living symbol.

The Great Mother most often appears to me in dreams as a croco-dile (it took me awhile to work that one out). In my conscious work, I engage with her energy in her deity form(s), but her archetype most often "teaches" me through the symbol of the crocodile. As Jung explained, the crocodile as a symbol can represent the living waters of the unconscious (Vedic thought also holds this as true), the soul, and the Great Mother archetype.

While the crocodile is the most common symbol my deep self serves up to communicate this specific energy complex, other ema-nations of form from the same complex sometimes arise, attempting to *make conscious* something my deep self wants me to know—something about which I am currently oblivious. I strongly encour-age you to track any symbol that appears to you over and over again. While the "dark waters" are by definition ambivalent at best, I have found them to be patient and kind, continuing to tell me the same thing over and over and over until I finally get it, understand it, and apply it.

It needs to be noted that the divine archetypes we will work with in this primer have already been made conscious and have been worked on and refined over an incredible span of time. So, in one sense, they are "flat" because there is general consensus about how to experience their information due to their use in myth, spiritual practice, and so on. That does not make them less numinous in the way they affect our deepest self.

Divine Archetypes: Profiles

When you work with divine archetypes for spiritual development, you'll want to invoke a deity whose archetypal energies are known and match up with the changes you seek. The Dalai Lama brought the concept of invoking the correct energetic antidote (or archetypal energy) into sharp focus in his teaching on the *Lam Rim Chen Mo* (*The Great Treatise on the Stages of the Path to Enlightenment*) at Lehigh University in

Pennsylvania in 2008.* He stressed repeatedly the need for precision when choosing "energetic medicine," such as a mantra or deity with which to engage, to ensure that the vibrational pattern offered is the remedy for what ails you. For example, if you sought a clear understanding of a teaching, you would meditate and use a mantra of Manjushri, the Buddha of knowledge and understanding. If instead you invoked Avalokiteshvara, the Buddha of compassion, you would not receive the same expansion of mental wisdom for which you were hoping.

To help you determine which divine archetypes best fit your particular needs, here we will explore a variety of deities who offer powerful support for spiritual development.

ROOT ARCHETYPES: DIVINE NATURE

In my opinion the divine spirits of nature are some of the oldest archetypes in our collective memory, and as time has gone on our remembering of them has become fuzzy. As a collective, we often find it easier to tune in to the deity or myth aspect of the archetype's energetic continuum. I like to picture the phenomenon as this: The nature-based aspect is like the root, the place from which the archetype sprouts, but it is buried out of sight. The deity aspect is like the bloom and easy to perceive.

One way to expand your knowledge of a specific archetype is to find out whether it had a specific plant associated with it, or what aspect of nature it expresses. For example, Crocus in Greek mythology was a human adolescent who had an unhappy relationship with a nymph. The gods took mercy on him and turned him into a plant that, even today, still bears his name: the crocus flower. As you read the profile below, you will see how the energy of the crocus flower heals discontent and disconnection. Studying this myth will round out your understanding of the Crocus Fairy archetype.

---

*The *Lam Rim Chen Mo* is a fifteenth-century Buddhist text on the stages of enlightenment.

Brigid is a goddess in Irish mythology who was known to be the patroness of the Moors. She is credited for bringing the fertility of early spring and also the energy to plant our ideas into the world. She was worshipped during Imbolc, a celebration marking the start of spring and representing the ability to learn from past mistakes, release that energy, and focus on new growth. She was revered by poets and thought to bring good cheer. Knowing these facets of Brigid's manifestation, you could in turn study any god or goddess associated with the Moors or with spring celebrations to help round out the archetype.

My point is that when you are drawn to a specific archetype, study as much of that energy complex as you can identify. Give yourself time as you do this; it is not something that can be rushed. Little by little a fuller picture will form. The reward for a thorough exploration is tremendous! When an archetypal image fully reveals itself to you, often it has already completed its work at the unconscious level. In other words, an aspect of your conscious self has already been altered in some way for your betterment. At this juncture the archetype that has mesmerized you often will lose its luster, and another that has work to do with you will take its place.

Goddess of the Marshlands

Catalyst for: Clearing confusion, misconceptions, and difficulties; giving rise to release and resurrection

Resonates with: Betel leaf, patchouli, frankincense, lemon

Working with the goddess of the marshlands can help you release chronic difficulties arising from past experiences that are stored in the unconscious mind and at a cellular level. Her energy expands your understanding in areas that were previously incomprehensible and brings to light the hidden fears and motives behind your actions. She holds the ability to not only understand but also release these experiences that have been holding you back from growth, helping you to see that they are in fact patterns of illusion and may be safely cleared.

In opening an internal channel, this goddess also unleashes a flowering of hidden talents and allows access to deep inner wisdom. This in turn allows you to connect with a clear understanding of personal truth that lights the next steps in your life path and grants you the inner strength to act upon this knowing.

Goddess of the Moors

Catalyst for: New ventures, ideas that transform lives and energize people, inspiration into action

Resonates with: Neroli, blood orange, cardamom

The goddess of the moors—those magical expanses of uncultivated grassy highlands—elevates the path to the heart, bringing courage and good cheer. Her stalwart energy does not allow you to be crushed by circumstances or to become dispirited, instead pushing you to spring back and arise with renewed confidence and faith that you can overcome whatever tries to put you down.

She offers the delightful gift of not taking yourself too seriously and grants the boon of the ability to relax and enjoy life, affirming your essential foolishness and allowing you to become more loving and let in the love that already surrounds you.

Acorn Dryad

Catalyst for: Process, overcoming struggle, reaching your goals

Resonates with: Galangal, vetiver, white lotus

This tiny but powerful dryad holds the energy to help you foster an idea all the way to maturation and develop patience and pleasure in process. Inviting her energy into your life will help you overcome procrastination and stagnation. Working with her energy rekindles the desire and motivation to go ahead with ideas and goals when the struggle seems too much.

Oak Dryad

Catalyst for: Stability, strength, channeling energy

Resonates with: Blue chamomile, patchouli, elemi

The energy of this dryad helps balance masculine energy between the poles of nurturing caregiver and heroic warrior, allowing you to find a point of equilibrium between stoic strength and self-care. Invoke him to help you access your own inner wisdom, or use his energy in conjunction with oracle tools such as tarot cards, runes, and so on. Call upon him for help in accessing all that you are so that you can complete your own personal hero/heroine's journey.

Weeping Willow Dryad

Catalyst for: Discernment, untangling, understanding

Resonates with: Pine, lime, lavender

Sometimes we find ourselves facing selfish or manipulative behaviors disguised as love, such as when friends or family are overly demanding, become emotionally needy, or seek attention through negative behavior or self-centeredness. In turn, we may become guarded or develop a prickly persona to keep these people at a distance.

Calling on this compassionate dryad can provide you with the energy you need to sever the cords holding you to this entangling mess. In the aftermath she transmutes this energy, providing the feeling of being safe and at peace, deep spiritual healing, and the ability to trust and open up again.

If you are the perpetrator of these behaviors, invoking her energy will allow you to practice selflessness, give love freely, respect the freedom and individuality of others, and practice emotional containment.

Crocus Fairy

Catalyst for: Harmony, partnership, love, cohesion, expression

Resonates with: Rose, vanilla, red spikenard

Invoking this fairy brings serenity, joy, and emotional stability. You can call on her energy to integrate all members of a family (or any close group) into a unit. She can be especially beneficial when a family is welcoming a new child but is also useful when a family begins to fray at the edges and unification is required. If family members are easily upset or moody, her energy will facilitate the release of these tensions. Her loving and protective energy opens and clears the emotional and mental bodies.

One of the special boons she offers is the ability to accept and become involved with the world and to share your unique talents. Under her auspices she dissolves the limiting energy of needless withdrawal, isolation, self-protection, fragility to the point of personal detriment, and the lack of inner strength to be fully in the world.

Dogwood Fairy

Catalyst for: Dreamscapes, rapid shifts in consciousness, magical understanding

Resonates with: Massoia bark, jasmine, Chinese rice flower

The energy of this ethereal being helps carry messages from your dream self to your waking self and allows you to navigate your inner and outer world. She expands intellectual knowledge until it reaches the exalted levels that dance on the border of the infinite so that it is no longer just knowledge, but magical understanding.

She also aids with a conscious sacrifice of self to a larger ideal and with shape-shifting all aspects of self.

Morning Glory Fairy

Catalyst for: Beneficial shifts, attaining more substance in your life, expressing a more authentic self

Resonates with: Agarwood, galangal, rosewood

The energy of this fairy guides the soul toward satisfying your true inner needs versus quelling the outer symptoms of an emotional problem or need with a stifling or dampening substance or energy. Her strong and supportive energy increases your willpower to break addiction in any manifestation, be it food, alcohol, excessive media, self-generated drama to distract from discontent, or any other expression.

Calling upon her energy will help you identify what you really are hungry for at a soul level and simultaneously eliminate the miasma of the unhealthy substitute. If you are overly susceptible to depression or despair due to fluctuating life events, or bouts of mania followed by depression, she can bring equilibrium and the ability to integrate suffering and joy into a positive whole.

Sunflower Fay

Catalyst for: Clarity, structure, fairness, balance

Resonates with: Black pepper, lemon, sandalwood

Inviting this fay into your life helps heal the energy around unequal treatment for any being, narcissism, and cruel or punitive behavior. She also brings the gift of valuing a point of view that differs from your own.

Working with this luminous energy helps you open to a radiant emotional life and to understanding the importance of the emotional body. She expands your ability to create order and organization, to experience moderation and personal discipline, to develop the left brain, and to appreciate and master the classical arts.

THE DARK GODDESS

The Dark Goddess can be seen in various manifestations in cultures around the world, always with similar traits and energies. She is the goddess of the unconscious; of the dissolution or undoing of things, which gives us the raw material to authentically reformat into a new way of being; of concern for the human condition; of addressing challenges and disharmonies by going inward to the cause instead of ascending away from them; of dealing with the aspects of self and life that are unpleasant. She is a loving goddess, but she can be frightening. She is the archetype whose energy we need when we are denying shadow/painful aspects of self and environment or wanting to wish away unpleasantness because it is too hard to deal with. The Dark Goddess shows us the way to deal with this energy. She also teaches the understanding of symbols, rituals, mystical traditions, and unconventional healing arts.

We often fear the power of the Dark Goddess—darkness, destruction, dissolution—but her energy is that of the dark moon, the harbinger of rebirth and the fire that burns in order to renew. Rob Preece explains this beautifully.

> In all deities, a dual nature is evident; light and dark, upper world and underworld, peaceful and wrathful. The forces of the Shadow are not inherently demonic and terrible. Light and dark, good and evil, creation and destruction are relative dualities that have no ultimate true nature. They are not absolutes. It is our ignorance and lack of insight that seeks out one and fears the other.
>
> The forces of the Shadow become demonic because they are not given appropriate recognition, conscious understanding, or respect. . . . In the East, the dark side of reality, with its potency, wildness, and destructiveness, is given the due respect it requires and placed in the temple as the wrathful deity, the bringer of wisdom and light.[2]

Following are some specific examples of Dark Goddess manifestations, as a foundation for exploration of her archetypal energy.

Palden Lhamo

Catalyst for: Psychic abilities, protection, deep magic, personal power

Resonates with: Betel leaf, red spikenard

In the Buddhist pantheon, Palden Lhamo is a wrathful deity, a fierce and powerful Dark Goddess, one of the eight guardians of the law (dharma), and the only female among them. In *The Psychology of Buddhist Tantra,* Rob Preece describes Palden Lhamo this way:

> She is a ferocious-looking crone, a wild and terrible demoness, riding a mule across an ocean of blood. She is the queen of witches and spirits, bringing them under her power. She scatters vile diseases on those who disregard her, or who act in ways that are malignant to the Dharma. She bestows psychic powers such as clairvoyance and a knowledge of healing. . . . Palden Lhamo has a lunar link, with her hair adorned by a moon, as though she is . . . the dark moon. This dark side of the feminine can clearly be seen as a Shadow to the light lunar forms, which White Tara most closely embodies.[3]

Palden Lhamo embodies the very important flip side of White Tara's energy. She is the Crone, the Dark Goddess, and the wildness within. Palden Lhamo is ready to help us recognize, root out, and transform the deepest, most disturbing aspects of self. She protects us from harm inflicted not only by others but also by ourselves. She teaches the value of the deep feminine gifts of healing and clairvoyance, and she manifests the death/rebirth forces of the dark moon. Her ultimate nature is as a protector of the way of compassion for self and others.

Lilith

Catalyst for: Thriving in your original nature

Resonates with: Betel leaf, White lotus

*The story goes that she demanded equality right from the
start. When Adam demanded that she be his "helpmate"
(i.e., slave), Lilith responded: "Why should I lie beneath
you, when I am your equal since both of us were created
from dust?"*

ARIEL GUTTMAN AND KENNETH JOHNSON,
MYTHIC ASTROLOGY APPLIED

Lilith is one of the most misunderstood archetypes of all time.
Historically she has been vilified for asking that her needs be met and
that she be valued for who she is, rather than who the people around
her would like her to be, and ultimately for standing up for herself.

Originally he and she, Adam and Lilith, were created equal and
together and set in the Garden of Eden to give things their names
and thereby bring the world into manifestation. They had a very
difficult time because Lilith insisted upon full equality, which
Adam refused, and they could not agree upon anything. Adam
would have sex with Lilith only if he was on top and she was on
the bottom because he was superior, having been created from
pure dust, and she was inferior, having come from filth and sediment. After some time Lilith realized that Adam was never going
to accept as valid and worthwhile anything she had to offer, so
she uttered the secret name of God, flew off, and vanished into
the air.[4]

Thus Lilith, mother to the world, was set in the Garden of Eden to
bring the world into manifestation. Though she was not to fulfill this
role in the Garden, later stories say that it was Lilith herself in the guise
of a serpent who helped Eve awaken.

Adam, her husband, her partner, her presumed love, told her continually that she was not good enough the way she was. Just sit with
that for a moment.

Lilith was labeled flawed and unworthy because she had come from filth and sediment (primal material). Yet sediment makes soil fertile, able to create and sustain life. Lilith was the fertile counterpart to the dry, barren dust from which Adam was made. The patriarchal telling of the story, however, distorts this aspect of the original human duality to categorize Lilith as sullied.

After rejecting Adam and leaving the Garden of Eden, Lilith had sex with "demons" and birthed many mystical progeny (which make our world a richer place to dwell). God then sent three angels to capture her—Senoy, Sansenoy, and Semangelof. The message from Adam and God was: if you don't come back and submit yourself, we will kill a hundred of your children every day. When Lilith would not give in to that kind of bullying, they countered with: then we will drown you.

Up to this point, the sum total of "rebellion" that Lilith had participated in was asking to be valued for who she was. When the powers that be demanded her subservience, she held strong against them. Lilith knew that submitting to Adam and agreeing that she was a lesser being would not be satisfactory to her on a deep level. On the other hand, coupling with water spirits, for example, and birthing "the sea of the unconscious, from which the feminine aspect of our wisdom arises from the depths of our psyche,"[5] provided an incredibly rich and wonderful gift for humankind.

Lilith shows us that being cut off from our soul and our sense of self-worth is to be cut off from our power, strength, and potential. This Dark Goddess helps us tap in to our anger and moral outrage. She reminds us that Mother Nature will orchestrate a forest fire when it is needed for healthy progression. After the fire, in the charred remains, there is breathing room for new green shoots instead of the dead, tangled, brittle undergrowth of a dying forest. You, too, may need to use great force to make way for new growth.

Lilith brings us to the brink of greatness of self and serves as a guide in the darkness. She gives us star eyes to burn in the darkness, the strength to be fierce and firm, and the vision of our own terrible beauty. She opens us to our own inner bravery until we find firm footing in our unique, perfect soul. Her energy is beautiful, seductive, independent, and perhaps frightening for some, as she is not controlled by outside forces but only by the dictates of her own heart. She listens solely to her own counsel and refuses to belong to anyone—mother, father, mate, society, or children. Her energy is that of pure possibility without restriction. Use this archetype to bring deeply passionate, free, feral feminine energy into your life.

Snake

Catalyst for: Authentic growth, growth through cycles, using potions to heal, transmutation, kundalini

Resonates with: Betel leaf (Dark Goddess/Snake); lemon (Athena)

Snake's energy is that of old knowledge and ancient wisdom, of matter becoming conscious. It is associated with the dynamic experience of radical awakenings and shifts in awareness that push us over a threshold, requiring us to never go back to an old way of being.

Snake appears in the Garden of Eden to direct Eve in her first shaky steps of awakening by encouraging her to eat of the fruit of the Tree of All Knowledge. Snake also plays a dramatic role as the hair of Medusa, a fascinating tale of kundalini pushing upward. Medusa, a Libyan Dark Goddess representing the dark moon mysteries, is the old guard of ancient Goddess wisdom. Athena's role in the slaying of Medusa allowed Athena to integrate Medusa's deep, almost unfathomable wisdom and make it readily available to humanity in many forms, including healing potions and the systematic knowledge required to make them usable.

These potions were made from the blood of Medusa's neck: blood from the right vein could cure and restore life, while the left vein gave forth blood that took life instantaneously. Athena gave this blood to Asclepius, the god of healing. His emblem was the caduceus, a winged staff encoiled by two snakes. The symbolism of the entwined snakes speaks to the melding of masculine and feminine energy and the integration of Medusa's wisdom. Patients would sleep at his temple overnight, and Asclepius would base their treatments upon the deep, hidden information made conscious through their dreams.

The gift of the very essence of these mystery rites, the blood of Medusa, which Athena awarded to Asclepius, in part symbolizes progress toward healing the cleft between male and female internally and externally and ultimately the push toward the unity of self—the alchemical marriage. Asclepius was one of the first healers to translate the deep mystery of the feminine into a more readily understandable form; in fact, the information needed to understand and organize the energetic and healing properties of essential oils is a direct result of this transference of information into our age.

The combined energies of Medusa, Athena, and Asclepius allowed for the integration of the second chakra energy (feminine, deep mysteries) of the Medusa era into the third chakra energy (masculine, logic) of "modern" society. Athena, a symbol of reason and left-brain organizational thought, slew Medusa but did not discard her energy. Instead, she translated and absorbed Medusa's primordial feminine power and wisdom, symbolized by placing Medusa's head, adorned with snakes, on the center of her aegis. Athena's breastplate was also fashioned with a depiction of Medusa's head, symbolizing the primordial feminine moving to the heart center through conscious understanding. Athena is surrounded by deep snake symbolism, reinforcing the truth that her function was not to quash the ancient feminine but rather to facilitate its evolution.

Although she is often depicted as the feminine trying to suppress self and adopt a masculine ethic, *Athena really embodies feminine energy becoming conscious to itself.* This is the story of kundalini energy pushing from the second to the third chakra.

Kundalini, or the serpent's power, will not be content to stop at this stage of our collective and personal evolution. She will continue winding her way through each one of our psychic learning centers (chakras), stimulating and exciting every cord of our being until she pushes us to our final release. The fourth chakra energy of loving compassion and expression will be the serpent's next destination in our collective growth journey.*

Snake's energy can be erotic, energizing, and crazy making. To authentically walk with the Dark Goddess or experience a sudden kundalini awakening at any level can be disorienting, frightening, shocking, and deeply felt. However, if we explore it with conscious and loving intent, such a radical opening inevitably leads to wisdom, fertility of self, radical growth, and intense beauty. We can use Snake's or Medusa's archetype to access the gifts of primordial wisdom and ancient magic, which will help us understand how to transform any state of being and balance the disorienting aspects.

POPULAR DEITIES OF MODERN CULTURE

Here are some divine archetypes with which you may be familiar, having heard their stories everywhere from your grandmother's knee to school to popular media. These deities have captured the collective imagination of modern culture—perhaps because their archetypal energy is so needed right now.

Pallas Athena

Catalyst for: Wisdom, intelligence, practicality, strategy

Resonates with: Lemon, black pepper, elemi, cardamom

Pallas Athena is the goddess of wisdom, justice, and handicrafts. She was born from her father Zeus's head (her mother was Metis,

---

*It is interesting to note that the Buddha Maitreya, the next Buddha to incarnate, is said to embody fourth chakra energy, and Shakyamuni, the historical Buddha, brought deep wisdom from the Void (ether) that he accessed under the bodhi tree when he reached enlightenment to the mental plane (third chakra) to teach a formerly unknown path. The evolution from the third to the fourth chakra mirrors the path we see in the West.

a primordial sea goddess).* Her parentage signifies one of her major roles: making profound wisdom conscious for practical use. She teaches creative visualization and how to harness natural laws so that you can manifest your ideas into the world for practical ends. For example, she taught civilization how to weave, how to make and use the rake and plow, and how to bridle a horse and yoke oxen. She bestows the gifts of strategy, foresight, planning, and understanding situations in their wholeness, which gives rise to success in business, political, academic, or scientific works. Call upon her for making your ideas reality and for finding the right action to bring about the intended results.

Hermes

Catalyst for: Crossing barriers within self, alchemical action, magic

Resonates with: Chinese rice flower, lavender, frankincense

Hermes is a psychopomp, or a guide of souls. He is one of the few gods that can freely travel between all realms—that is, Olympus, Earth, and Hades.† He rules boundaries between states of consciousness; one of his symbols is the herm, a square stone pillar often embedded in the earth at doorways, crossroads, and property lines and denoting a shift into a new energy or state. He revels in his role as the trickster, and his energy can jar you greatly, forcing a new perspective; as he leads the mind ever upward, you can access the magical sage—the alchemical aspect—of his nature. Call upon him to deliver messages from your dreams to your waking life, a connection that can deepen your ability to solve mundane problems and larger issues. Connecting your upper and lower worlds to your everyday life allows you to shift perspective and act upon this

---

*As we have discussed, the primordial sea is analogous to the collective unconscious, a place of vast wisdom that is not easy to access, as the mind cannot will this information to reveal itself.

†These realms can be understood as spirit (Olympus), everyday life (Earth), and the unconscious (Hades).

shift with quicksilver (mercurial) speed. Hermes also brings a sense of playfulness, the ability to take stock of yourself and adapt your behavior accordingly, not taking yourself too seriously, and he brings good fortune at the crossroads of life.

Venus

Catalyst for: Love, beauty, sensuality, the urge to fulfill creative desires*

Resonates with: Rose, blood orange, jasmine

Venus, the goddess of love and beauty, represents not only the principle of physical beauty but also the beauty within that radiates out. Different cultures and time periods have had different definitions of what beauty is; the energy of Venus transcends these categorizations and allows each person's unique beauty to shine. This energy makes a person truly intoxicating. Venus also governs art forms that are beautiful for beauty's sake. A plastic molded chair, for example, is very functional and will get the job done, but it is a far cry from a hand-bent willow chair. The latter requires the artisan to seek out each individual branch, feeling into its characteristics to visualize how it will mesh with each other branch, and finally with passion and love create the finished chair. It is easy to sense how different each chair feels. Both offer seating, but one is easily discarded while the other treasured. Venus rules passions that need not be rooted in the mundane. You may call upon this goddess to give the most sublime aspects of yourself to another or to invite their energy at this level into your life. She can also help you enjoy life on Earth with a sense of wonder and delight.

Pan

Catalyst for: Body wisdom, play, being grounded in self and nature

---

*It is interesting to note that both sensuality and creativity are born from the waters of the second chakra. One of Venus's creation stories holds that Zeus castrated his father and tossed his genitals into the sea, creating a white foam from which Venus was born as an adult goddess.

Resonates with: Vetiver, patchouli, vanilla, pink pepper seed

Pan is the primordial god of Earth, the wilds, and sexuality. He has never had a temple dedicated to him; instead grottoes, clear lakes, meadows, woods, and caves are his places of worship. His gift is helping us remember body wisdom so that we can get out of our heads and back into our instinctual selves.*

When you feel overwhelmed by life and yearn for simplicity, nature, quiet, and solitude, call upon Pan. His consorts are nymphs (nature spirits), and this dynamic brings playfulness and sexual intoxication that looses us from all bonds of the ordinary and sets us free in spiritual ecstasy so that we can let go completely and experience oneness. An invocation of Pan is truly a prayer to the divine.

Iris

Catalyst for: Self-care, kindness, forgiveness

Resonates with: Neroli, pine, rosewood

Iris is the daughter of the sea god Thaumas and the sea nymph Electra. She travels on a rainbow made of light and water between heaven and earth, delivering messages from the gods to earth and taking the prayers from mortals to the heavens. Everywhere she goes, she sows the energy of harmony through kindly communication. As a water goddess she invites you into the realm of emotions. How do you feel? Are you happy? Do you behave in a kind manner? Are your inner needs being met? She takes you deep into your own heart for healing and contentment. This is the practice of self-care. Once you have opened a radiant space in your heart, you can radiate your happiness and fulfillment back out into the world, and difficulties melt away. In this way Iris also brings the gift of forgiveness and being magnanimous. Ask Iris to deliver sincere messages from your

---

*Deepak Chopra often advises that when we cannot think our way out of a situation, we should ask our body, because it never lies. He claims that it cannot.

heart to those with whom you have discordant energy that you wish to heal.

The Moirae (Fates)

Catalyst for: Fulfilling your destiny

Resonates with: All the essential oils listed in this book; choose the one(s) that support the nexus where fate has guided you

The Moirae are beings of destiny, three wizened crones who spin and weave your future and, when the time is correct, cut the thread of your life. Destiny is often confusing; as it is being constructed, it is hard to see the horizon. Take heart, for this is a time of initiation. Initiation is one of those concepts that seems exciting on paper but often in reality gives you the sensation of awakening to your next steps as a trial by fire. Calling on the Moirae for clarity in your next steps will help lead you on your way. Remember that a large part of destiny is being able to choose actions in a nonreactive way. It is important to stay grounded (vetiver, patchouli), to keep a clear head and nimble mind (lemon, black pepper), and to go with the flow and make decisions moment to moment to best craft your reality (red spikenard, frankincense, massoia bark). If you must experience a loss before you can achieve a gain, take the time to really experience your emotions and mourn if needed (lavender). Working with the Fates will allow you to stay centered amid challenging situations and bring trust for the future and the unfolding of right action.

Ganesha

Catalyst for: Wisdom, excelling in your craft, receiving blessings

Resonates with: Rose, sandalwood, blue chamomile

Ganesha, perhaps the most beloved god of India, is part man (his body) and part elephant (his head), and he is the patron of sciences, arts, and creative activities. He is depicted as a jolly, rotund god who loves sweets and offering boons. Ganesha is also a remover of obstacles; you can call upon him to remove obstacles that may block your path and pave the way with blessings before you undertake any activity.

He aids the mind in perceiving circumstances and surroundings as a gestalt. He promotes open-mindedness and positive boundaries, and he helps you take inventory of your personal reality, with the intent to understand your behaviors and how they could be detracting from your full involvement with life.

Ganesha's mount is a clever mouse or rat that is able to understand small details and to pass anywhere. This energy denotes the specialization of a skill, the ability to deconstruct something and understand it in detailed parts, as well as the ability to learn about the world around you through your own observations and to thrive in varied environments.

3

Tattvas

Connecting with the Five Great Elements

Creation takes place due to the tattwas and by them it is sustained.

LORD SHIVA, IN *SHIVA SWARODAYA*

If a person is not earth, not water,
Not fire, not wind, not space,
Not consciousness, and not all of them,
What person is there other than these?

NAGARJUNA, *PRECIOUS GARLAND*

In this primer we will explore the primordial building blocks of reality, the Five Great Elements, known as the *tattvas* or *tattwas,* and humankind's relationship with them. The five tattvas are earth, water, fire, air/wind, and ether/space.

The foundational principle for this exploration is that the commonly known universe and its inhabitants, including the human race, animals, plants, and minerals, are all created by and sustained by the tattvas, although ultimately we are not them and cannot be confined and manipulated by them without our personal permission. The goal of this book is to unravel this seemingly paradoxical theory and make it accessible to all as a powerful tool for personal transformation and liberation.

Many of us wrestle with a fundamental question long asked by philosophers, artists, and spiritual seekers: What are we really made of? The goddess Isis received the "great secret" of the projection of matter (our elemental natures, the elemental nature of the world around us, and how it is organized) from the fallen angel Amnael. Plato found that "space [ether] is like a nurse to the whole cosmic order."[1] Maya Tiwari, an ayurvedic specialist, writes, "We are the air, water, soil, and light of this planet. Every grain of sand, every mountain range, every river, and every leaf contain the same elements. We celebrate nature in our very nature."[2] The Who mused about it in their music, and in my favorite lyrical expression of the subject, musicians Kate Bush and Moby claim, "We may live on in comets and stars"[3] and "We are all made of stars."[4]

According to many ancient philosophical systems, including ayurveda, they are right. Vedic wisdom teaches that everything in existence (within and without) is fashioned from the tattvas. We are all made of stars, waterfalls, flowers, sunshine, and every other substance in the universe, because we share these common constituents. This is the macrocosm-microcosm relationship: as above, so below.

Our common tattvic nature allows us to use the resonant energy of archetypal patterns to shape our inner and outer worlds. It is the basis of the elegantly simple practice of using essential oils and vibrational essences to affect the very fabric of our being—our elemental makeup—and the vibrant living world around us. The tattvas flavor our expression as individuals; their presence affects everything from the color and shape of our eyes to our intellect and emotional temperament. In the context of the tattvas, we can explore who we are, what we are made of, what that really means, and how we can use this understanding to live our most potent lives.

Becoming aware of the tattvas, their traits, and how they impact our self and our environment opens the door to a state of conscious self-direction. We achieve this self-directed state by focusing on the following tenets.

✦ Our personal characteristics—what we recognize as our bodies, thoughts, behaviors, and emotions—arise due to personal elemental combinations (i.e., which tattvas are more or less dominant in our makeup). Our personal tattvic arrangements are based on past causation patterns (karma).

✦ We have the ability to recognize our tattvic arrangements and to understand the ways in which the Five Great Elements have collated to form the basis of our behaviors.

✦ We have the ability to skillfully use this information to *consciously craft self.*

✦ We can actively address the unconscious, emotional body, and mental body and arrest unhealthy causation patterns that manipulate self.

✦ We can use essential oils and vibrational tools for personal betterment by directing their energy to balance our tattvic arrangment, until we are able to transcend the elements altogether.

The methodology we will explore allows us to directly access the deepest, most chthonic (primordial and hidden) aspects of self, the very energetic causation patterns that set all behaviors and thoughts into motion, *the very root of our existence!* The tattvas are the energy that drive archetypal patterns. They animate each chakra and cause our *doshas* (physical-energetic constitutional types) to form. They are the energetic skeletal structure that creates and sustains every aspect of our human existence. In understanding how each tattva operates and behaves, we can recognize their influence; by understanding how to access and work with them, we can ultimately free ourselves from any manipulation of free will and direct all of our self toward correcting the causation patterns of these elements.

As Mahayana philosopher Nagarjuna (ca. 150–250 CE) reminds us, we are not the Five Great Elements, nor, as the Heart Sutra says, anything other than them. Ultimately we are empty beings—on a very base level, we have the freedom to arrange our self into any pattern of behavior. We have no set inherent traits, only layered-on energy that makes up our unique energetic portrait, which in turn dictates how we look, feel, and act.

In the quest for energetic or karmic healing, we do not have to wait to be "reborn" by physically dying and taking rebirth. The theory and processes described here explore the possibility of experiencing many small deaths to ways of being, leading to rebirths of new patterns in this life. These shifts in consciousness are associated with understanding and changing the causation patterns (karma) that manipulate self by either keeping us ensnared in unhealthy energy or propelling us forward without awareness.

This combination of study and practice supports the conscious development of bridges between all aspects of self, allowing us to deliberately steer our personal destiny and, in due course, to fulfill personal dharma and be all that we were intended to be.

Every tradition has a slightly different take on how each tattva organizes and presents. Even among geographically close Eastern systems such as Hinduism, Shavism, Bon, Tibetan Buddhism, and other schools of Buddhism, there is variation on how each of these great elements is believed to operate and impact our reality. Tibetan lama Kalu Rinpoche spoke to the jumble of information that exists within even the same traditions.

> Any one of these various cosmologies is completely valid for the beings whose karmic projections cause them to experience their universe in that way. There is a certain relativity in the way one experiences the world. This means that all the possible experiences . . . are based upon karmic inclinations and degrees of individual development. Thus, on a relative level, any cosmology is valid. On an ultimate level, no cosmology is absolutely true.[5]

I have taken strands from each of these schools of thought, simplified them, and woven the threads together to achieve the whole that

I am presenting here. I look for truths that transcend the bounds of a single dogmatic thought system. My goal is to present an accessible system that makes these timeless truths readily available for personal use.

As Above, So Below:
The Macro/Microcosm

The infinitesimal magnitude of change evolves endlessly as we exchange our atoms and molecules with all the elements around us. While we bask in the sun, that solar energy becomes part of our being; when we walk through a forest, the trees and moisture and the god-filled black earth become part of our energy field. Our field of energy and that of the forest and the sun are identical.

MAYA TIWARI, *AYURVEDA: A LIFE OF BALANCE*

As mentioned before, there are several philosophies concerning the properties of the tattvas before they drop into form here on Earth. This book, however, will examine the tattvas as we experience them through the senses—sound (ether), touch (air), sight (fire), taste (water), and scent (earth)—and how they affect the human emotional, spirit, and mental bodies and the soul.

By understanding and experiencing the elemental microcosm, we can become fully aware of, and can work with, the macrocosm. The same patterns are reproduced at all levels of the cosmos, from the largest scale (macrocosm or universal level) down to the smallest scale (microcosm or metaphysical level). When we stimulate an exterior environment (macrocosm), it stirs our personal interior (microcosm). When we stimulate our personal interior (microcosm), it ripples out and affects the universe (macrocosm). Once we understand the resonant energies involved, we can use them to affect matter both internally and externally.

The intent in employing the five tattvas to consciously work with the subtle self is to free ourself from the manipulation of causation patterns* and restore our cellular memory of the "all-thing."

Tiwari notes:

> According to the Rishis, from pure consciousness arose the sound of OM. In turn, the Five Great Elements took birth. These five elements take the form, in the human body, of the three doshas, or bodily humors. It is from these doshas that our individual constitution . . . is formed. As we come to identify ourselves with these primal elements, we create a bridge that allows us to climb back to the sky: we approach our cosmic roots.[6]

Tattvas and Vibrational Energy

The word *tattva* can be translated as "thatness," which can be further understood as the essence that creates the feeling of existence. Swami Satyasangananda tells us:

> In the *Tantraraja Tantra,* Shakti asks Shiva, "Where do all the tattwas exist, in the body or out of it?" Shiva replies that the tattwas permeate the entire body and mind. Everything you do and think is under the influence of these tattwas. Therefore . . . it is necessary to understand how the tattwas behave and in which manner they can be controlled and utilized.[7]

The five tattvas, like all other forms in the universe, arise from vibration. So "the essence which creates the feeling of existence" or inherent self is just a label describing emanations of form that helps us

---

*A causation pattern defines the relationship between two events in which the second event is a direct consequence of the first. In our exploration, a causation pattern refers to a calcified energetic network or path from which reflexive behaviors arise; the event that calcifies the energetic network (the cause) leads to the reflexive behavior (the effect).

interpret the concepts of self and environment. For example, what we refer to as the tattva *earth* does not mean just "dirt" but is to be understood also as a combination of light and vibrational patterns that have collated to "act like" a specific set of behaviors. So we experience this tattva as the earth around us but as the same time it is a set of behaviors that arise internally.

The ironic aspect of working with the tattvas as a system is that we do not want to be ensnared and bound by them. As Shiva stated, it is necessary to understand how they behave so they can be controlled and utilized. As all things manifest in dualism, there are positive and negative aspects to each of the five tattvas. Our personal elemental arrangements manipulate our existence by constantly interacting with external resonant factors, which stimulate and then set behavioral patterns into motion. A major focus of meditation, breath work, and sound work in many traditions is to become "one who has gone beyond the elements"—one who has awakened, or in Jungian terms, achieved individuation. But to do so, we must engage with and purify the patterns that are associated with each element.

In the Vedic tradition, the tattvas manifest as a series in which each successive element derives from its predecessor and inherits a heavier (slower) vibration.

+ The first element to evolve is ether, also called *akasha*. Ether is *undifferentiated matter,* which contains an infinite amount of potential energy. It is the subtle state in which both energy and matter exist in their dormant potential state at the heart of consciousness.

+ As the energy inherent in the particles of akasha begins to vibrate, movement is stimulated and the element air emerges. Because the particles of air have the greatest freedom of movement, the air element is seen as *all-pervading motion.*

+ The excessive energy that the movement of air creates stimulates the emergence of the next element, fire. There is less movement in the fire element than in the air element; it is seen primarily as *light*. As Satyasangananda says, "This tattva is energy in its first stage of manifestation, when it is primarily conceived as light. It is by the appearance of light that form is perceived. In the absence of light there is no form which can be perceived."[8] The ego also comes into being here.

+ With decreasing motion, the fire element condenses into the water element. The energy of the water element is to pervade, and it can be understood as *intensely active matter* that, having begun to emerge out of the fire element, is confined within a definite space and moves within a small radius, although it has not broken into specific forms yet.

+ The final element evolves from a further decrease in vibration that causes water to solidify into earth, which appears *static*.

Tattvas, Chakras, and Doshas

The tattvic, or elemental, energies, representing the most primal aspects of self, give rise to the more refined chakral energies within the self, which in turn manifest as the doshas and their associated characteristics. Understand your energies, understand your toolbox, and your life will be infinitely richer.

The relationship between the tattvas and their correlating chakras offers an interesting study. The tattvas manifest the denser primal vibration that is the heart of the evolving energy expressed in the more complex pattern at each chakra center. As you read the profiles of each, pay special attention to how similar the profiles are but how the energy blooms into a more complex pattern from element to chakra. This is not to say that one is better than another; they are equally important, and the true wisdom comes from knowing when to invoke one or the other.

Doshas in the ayurvedic tradition are the three basic metabolic principles connecting body, mind, and spirit. Each dosha arises from two elements, and a person's dosha profile dictates his or her behavior and body type.

+ **Kapha:** This dosha is responsible for body mass, structure, and fluids. Kapha is archetypal Mother Earth energy. A kapha type tends to be nurturing, gentle, and fertile, with a strong emotional IQ and sexual energy. This type is curvaceous, with large, liquid eyes and thick hair, and is ruled by the food body (the first layer of the material self). Its function is to restore our cosmic memory. Kapha traits are oily, dense, cool, heavy, stable, and smooth. The tastes inherent to this type are sweet, sour, and salty.

+ **Pitta:** This dosha is responsible for metabolism, digestive acids, and enzymes. A pitta type tends to have vast intelligence and energy, ambition, and aggression. This type is athletic, with a strong and toned body, and is ruled by the mind body (the third layer of the material self). Its function is to govern will and desires and makes the whole of the cosmos visible to us—what we understand as imagination, ideas, and visions and our ability to project what we conjure into the world. Pitta traits are hot, oily, light, intense, and fluid. The tastes inherent to this type are sour, pungent, and salty.

+ **Vata:** This dosha is responsible for spatial cavities in the body. Vata types tend to have an innate innocence and seek a spiritual life, not being concerned with earthly rules, and they have the shortest karmic slack* of all the dosha types. This type is thin, with protruding joints, dry skin, and curly or kinky hair, and is ruled by prana (the second layer of the material self). Its function is to feed *ahamkara* (the center of individual, mental, emotional, psychic, and physical functioning). All of our past, present, and future is stored here, and from this space comes our need to paint, sing, write, dance, procreate, worship, explore, ask questions, find

---

*In other words, vatas feel the repercussions of their actions quickly and deeply.

answers, have relationships, and so on. Vata traits are dry, cold, light, mobile, erratic, and rough. The tastes inherent to this type are bitter, astringent, and pungent.

Though every one of us contains within us all five elements and all the dosha types, the average person generally has two dosha types that predominate. You might, for example, be a kapha-vata type or a pitta-vata type. Very rarely is a person truly tridoshic.

ELEMENT	CHAKRA*	DOSHA
Ether	Fifth (vishuddha)	Vata
Air	Fourth (anahata)	Vata
Fire	Third (manipura)	Pitta
Water	Second (svadhishthana)	Kapha, pitta
Earth	First (muladhara)	Kapha

*In the next chapter we will explore the seven main chakras. You may wonder why only five are represented here. The sixth chakra (ajna) is formed from all the elements combined. The seventh chakra (sahasrara) is beyond the elements. Neither the sixth nor the seventh chakra has a dosha correlation.

Tattvas and Their Symbols:
Shapes and Colors

Thubten Chodron, a Tibetan Buddhist nun, explains why the elements organize into specific arrangements to teach us, using the example of why fully enlightened beings, such as Buddhas who are depicted on stupas as the five elements, could emanate in any configuration and choose specific colors and shapes to help guide us.

They need a way to communicate with us to lead us on the path out of suffering to full enlightenment. Since we are embodied beings who relate to color, shape, and other objects of the senses, the compassionate Buddhas appear in various forms in order to communicate with us. . . . Each deity is a manifestation of the same enlightened qualities—love, compassion, joy, equanimity, generosity, ethical discipline, patience, enthusiasm, concentration, and wisdom—although each manifestation may emphasize a particular quality. For example, Tara symbolizes enlightened activity. . . . If we think about the qualities of a Buddha, how would those qualities look if they appeared in color, shape, and form? Even though all Buddhas have the same internal traits and qualities, they appear in different manifestations to emphasize certain characteristics. For example, an artist or a musician has an internal feeling or meaning he wants to express. In order to communicate it, he draws a picture with color and shape . . . to express what's going on inside. In a similar way, Buddhas express their realizations in different external forms.[9]

The concept of "consciousness" organizing into specific shapes and colors (including plants, minerals, and metals) to stimulate the human process of awakening is not as developed in the West, but it is not ignored. Jung explored this concept in depth, and a fascinating study emerged from the Expressionist art movement with painters such as Matisse, Klee, and Kandinsky. Matisse, in fact, declared that colors act like a "cerebral sedative."[10]

The Eastern art form of mandalas uses sacred geometry and color "maps" to lead its makers to enlightenment. Buddhist scholar Giuseppe Tucci describes a mandala as follows:

Each of its colors reflected components of the human personality, the poisons blocking the way: white reflected ignorance, yellow pride, red lust, green jealousy and blue-black anger. There was no doubt that this imagery was a support for learning and meditation. It helped the disciple, led by a "guru," to bring light within the labyrinth of consciousness those "obscuring passions" that had to be driven out. The colors are points of reference, a system of signs, a carefully chosen grammar for reshaping the personality.[11]

The Tibetan Buddhist tradition teaches that

on what we may call the level of archetypes, a stupa incorporates five basic geometric shapes corresponding to the five elements— earth, water, fire, air and space—out of which the world and all the atoms within it are composed. Furthermore, the overall shape of a stupa bears a close resemblance to the image of a seated Buddha . . . . *Merely by viewing such harmoniously balanced images,* we receive subtle benefit, experienced as a feeling of peace, well-being and wholeness. Finally, it should be noted that the various levels of the stupa correspond to the various levels of the spiritual path culminating in full enlightenment.[12]

It is clear that no matter what school of thought you prescribe to, there is a common consensus that "merely by viewing such harmoniously balanced images, we receive subtle benefit," allowing us to work with aspects of self that are so chthonic that the linear mind is not capable of accessing them without assistance. If we stay on task and work with tattvic and other vibrational tools in earnest, we will ultimately support the full liberation of self.

Tattvas: Profiles

Nature is not improved save through its own nature.

ARISLEUS

To fully understand the healing vibration offered by an essential oil, it is imperative not only to understand the oil's profile (see chapter 6), but also to understand the vibration that gave rise to its elemental arrangement. For example, galangal is earth with the seed of water; this combination of elements gives rise to galangal's pattern of being in synchronicity (water/flow) and being able to benefit from circumstances (earth/gain). To gain a well-rounded understanding of galangal's properties, you would first read the profiles of its constituent tattvas (listed on pages 52–60) and then read the essential oil profile.

If you were exploring an essential oil not profiled in this book, you would have to research the plant from which the oil is distilled. Most ayurvedic textbooks list the effects of various plants on the doshas, or you can simply identify the plant's predominant tastes—sweet, pungent, sour, et cetera. If you are familiar with the system, you can work it backward, because all of those traits are produced by the tattvas. For example, earth and water create kapha, and kapha's energy is sweet. So you can know that a plant listed as having a sweet taste is produced from the tattvas earth and water. You can then also read about the behavior of the plant (its physical, mental, and spiritual actions) to see how the tattvas are reflected within that framework, and you can read about which deities or animals a plant might be associated with through cultural and mythological history. With that deeper exploration you can begin to identify how a specific plant and its essential oil might resonate with a particular tattva and archetypal energy and begin to weave together all the disparate details into a whole. (When you're doing the research, I would recommend reading about a plant from multiple sources, because plants have a wide spectrum of actions and associations, and most books only offer a snapshot of each one.)

It is important to remember that you yourself are made from the same elements as the essential oils, and it is this commonality that creates the resonant bridge that allows you to access and be reformatted by the vibrational patterns they offer. This sentiment is beautifully reflected in the Chandogya Upanishad, an ayurvedic root text: "The essence of all beings is Earth. The essence of the Earth is Water. The essence of Water is plants. The essence of plants is the human being."

ETHER

The vibration of this tattwa is said to be so subtle that it cannot be perceived by the external senses. Our senses have not been tuned to that frequency; therefore, as long as we function through them, we cannot experience the subtle vibration of akasha or ether.

SWAMI SATYASANGANANDA

We come spinning out of nothingness, scattering stars like dust.

RUMI

Sanskrit Name: Akasha

Location: Throat

Chakra Correlation: Fifth (vishuddha, inner muse)

Color: Black

Sacred Geometry: Oval

Sacred Syllable: *Ham*

Key Traits: Expansion, diffusion, timelessness—the convergence of the past, present, and future. Limitlessness, the void, an absence of light, described as black or transparent—within this blackness all the colors of creation exist. The space of consciousness that is located in front of the closed eyes (*chidakasha*). Ether is everything and nothing—All into One. At the level of the mind, ether is said to control the emotions and passions in humankind (*control*, not *generate*) and to turn one away from sensorial experiences. It is auspicious for spiritual work and contraindicated for material gain (birthing or the accumulation of gross matter). Without conscious cultivation, ether is active or dominant in the average individual for only five minutes per hour.

Gifts

+ Opens you to spiritual gifts such as clairvoyance, clairaudience, and being a clear channel—all information beyond the rational mind
+ Teaches and promotes the highest expression of self, understanding truth, and expressing that personal understanding as a lifestyle
+ Fosters true creativity
+ Grants an understanding of gestalts, symbolism, myth, and subtle information
+ Encourages good communication skills: expressing clearly what you mean and feel, along with the ability to really hear what others say, including what is left unsaid

Shadow Issues

Too little ether:

+ Feeling contracted and immutable
+ Lacking spiritual connection and the ability to transcend the physical world
+ Difficulty recognizing and expressing your own truth
+ Difficulty with communication: not hearing what others are saying or not saying what you mean

Too much ether:

+ Feeling spaced out and disoriented, afraid of being alone or lost

AIR

Vayu tattwa, like its cause, akasha tattwa, is invisible in the material sense. At this subtle stage, matter is still in its undifferentiated form. It can be described as energy in motion. Constant motion creates change, and, therefore, the influence of vayu tattwa causes instability and fickleness in a person and the environment.

SWAMI SATYASANGANANDA

Your task is not to seek for love, but merely to seek and find all the barriers within yourself that you have built against it.

RUMI

Sanskrit Name: Vayu

Location: Spiritual heart

Chakra Correlation: Fourth (anahata/heart)

Color: Smoky green

Sacred Geometry: Circle

Sacred Syllable: *Yam*

Key Traits: Gaseous in form; has the nature of wind; represents kinetic energy in all forms—electrical, chemical, vital, and so on. Air is the breath of life. It is the prana that allows us to be animated and vital. It expresses movement through contraction and expansion. It also creates instability and restlessness, so it is not helpful for material gain. The air element is responsible for unanticipated insights; it is an auspicious element to invoke while creating original work.

Gifts

+ Carries and facilitates positive change; relates to the intuitive body
+ Promotes curiosity, learning, and flexibility on all levels
+ Allows the mind to achieve new insight and fresh perspectives
+ Associates with abstract understanding and dreaming; air is the element of active dreamers—the visualization of what could be
+ Promotes freedom from attachments (dogmatic, emotional, etc.)
+ Supports shifting and directing consciousness and swiftness in all forms

+ Bridges the mundane and the divine to foster love of all types, forgiveness, and compassion

Shadow Issues

Too little air:

+ Constricted heart center, leading to a tendency to hold grudges and an inability to give or receive love, resulting in a dismal view of life
+ No personal intuition

Too much air:

+ Disturbs the mind, causing difficulty concentrating, thinking things through, or sitting for meditation
+ The inability to finish projects, scattered energy, and jitteriness
+ Poor internal anchoring; being overly swayed by environmental factors

FIRE

The birth of form is closely connected with the birth of ego. We know that ego identifies with form, which results in attachment. Therefore, without the presence of form there can be no attachment. So we have to understand agni tattwa, not just as the first manifestation of form, but also as the stage when ahamkara, which has been developing simultaneously, becomes aware of something outside itself for the first time. Thus the germ of individual ego is born.

SWAMI SATYASANGANANDA

Even after all this time
The sun never says to the earth, "You owe me."
Look what happens with
A love like that,
It lights the whole sky.

HAFIZ

Sanskrit Name: Agni

Location: Solar plexus/navel

Chakra Correlation: Third (manipura/inner sun)

Color: Dull red

Sacred Geometry: Triangle

Sacred Syllable: *Ram*

Key Traits: Energy in the first stages of manifestation, primarily perceived as light; birth of the "I" self, or ego. This element's red color denotes extreme heat; it is a consuming, devouring force that can be unstable and destructive. It can also be understood as a catalyst for change, growth, evolution, and increase. This element's actions are unbiased in application toward specific quadrants of life; its primary function is to restructure. Fire is the catalyst in life. It is the great transformer that consumes to renew.

Gifts

+ Instills the capacity to initiate projects on every level, passion, enthusiasm, and warmth
+ Promotes the ability to transmutate any situation that does not serve your highest self
+ Supports the birth of personal ego—experiences centered in personal identity
+ Relates to the mental body, the ability to direct personal will, and the need to directly act upon ideas in the physical world
+ Supports the energy of the divine masculine (protector and champion)
+ Provokes sensations of bliss, growth, change, increase, and evolution

Shadow Issues

Too little fire:

+ Inability to stand up for yourself or deal with confrontation
+ Passivity

Too much fire:

+ Arrogance, self-centered attitude, feeling superior; being dominating or believing "my way is the only way"
+ Lack of self-control, volatile expression of self, instability, childishness
+ "Hot" issues: anger, being quarrelsome and confrontational

WATER

Apas, or water, is derived from the root aap, *which means "to pervade." Apas tattwa can be described as a vast quantity of intensely active matter which has begun to emerge out of agni tattwa. It is matter that has not yet been broken up into cohesive and separate bodies, because the atoms and molecules reverberating within this tattwa are still in a state of chaos. It is said that the physical universe is arranging itself in apas tattwas before its emergence, hence the term "pregnant waters," alluding to the idea of the universe contained within the womb of apas.*

SWAMI SATYASANGANANDA

Soul serves as a cup for the juice that leaves the intellect in ruins.

RUMI

Sanskrit Name: Apas

Location: Pelvic bowl

Chakra Correlation: Second (svadhishthana/chalice of self)

Color: Silver

Sacred Geometry: Recumbent crescent moon

Sacred Syllable: *Vam*

Key Traits: Energy at this stage is still barely perceivable and contains within it matter about to be birthed; therefore, it has a more creative influence on worldly matters. Water is the great gateway to all things hidden—the emotions, subconscious, and unconscious. This element is always reforming itself into new arrangements, so results from the water element are not permanent. It is used to birth new environments.

Gifts

+ Feelings, rhythm, understanding natural cycles, the unconscious, and the emotional body
+ "Pregnant waters," pervasiveness, creativity, receptivity—allowing self to be filled
+ Expression of emotional states—the ability to thaw/release frozen emotions (ice/steam), whether clean, murky, or salty (tears)
+ Rebirth and renewal, empathy, fluidity
+ Supporting alignment with synchronistic events; grace
+ The dream and soul medium—allows you to actively access and work with the collective unconscious and use dreams for personal growth
+ Divine feminine—working with and understanding all that the divine feminine holds
+ Feeling contentment not determined by outside circumstances

Shadow Issues

Too little water:

+ Emotionally desolate; lacking empathy
+ Internally brittle, in need of soul or emotional nourishment
+ Unable to work with or understand dreams

✦ Relying on external circumstances to create feelings of contentment

Too much water:

✦ Consumed by and drowning in emotion; being emotionally tempestuous
✦ Using escapism to avoid life

EARTH

The last tattwa in the matter/energy complex is prithvi, or earth. Prithvi is also known as bhumi, which means "to be" or "to exist." It also means the ground and earth we live upon, which signifies existence. In prithvi tattwa, the particles of energy have been condensed until they appear almost static, rotating only within the immediate space surrounding each atom. Thus, in this tattwa, energy appears as concrete matter.

SWAMI SATYASANGANANDA

Let the beauty you love be what you do. There are a thousand ways to kneel and kiss the earth.

RUMI

Sanskrit Name: Prithvi

Location: Base of the spine/coccyx

Chakra Correlation: First (muladhara/root)

Color: Matte yellow

Sacred Geometry: Square

Sacred Syllable: *Lam*

Key Traits: Energy at this stage vibrates at much lower and denser rates and is associated with solidity, weight, cohesion, and gain. Earth is the means to create foundation and structure in our lives. This is the element to invoke for material gain and permanence in every aspect, including physical and mental stability (long-term memory, feeling emotionally stable, etc.) and your environment. It is contraindicated for situations of being in a rut, feeling stuck, or any stagnation.

Gifts

+ Stability, security, being grounded
+ Healing discord in family lineage and DNA
+ Determination, patience, endurance, practicality, positive parenting
+ Acquisition, increase and creating abundance, practicing generosity
+ Devic communication, having a "green thumb," preparing nutritious meals

Shadow Issues

Too little earth:

+ Being ungrounded, being unable to accumulate wealth, or having resources slip through your fingers
+ Feeling uneasy in your body; not enjoying the sensual pleasures of being on this earth

Too much earth:

+ Plodding, heavy, dull, slow, greedy, gluttonous
+ Feeling stuck, lacking creativity, being overly pragmatic
+ Being stubborn, entrenched in a way of being, only believing what you can understand with the sense organs

4
Chakras

Keeping Vital Energy Flowing

Each chakra is constituted of one basic element. Within mooladhara is prithvi (earth) tattwa; in swadhishthana, apas (water) tattwa; in manipura, agni (fire) tattwa; in anahata, vayu (air) tattwa; in vishuddhi, akahsa (ether) tattwa. The particular element which governs each chakra indicates the level at which the chakra vibrates and operates.

Our entire range of consciousness, thoughts and actions is governed by the activities of these chakras. . . . As long as they are not fully activated, we are limited in every action and experience . . . these chakras are directly influenced by concentration on each tattwa.

Swami Satyasangananda

Though the body appears to be a material object, in reality it's a field of energy, transformation, and intelligence. When we look beyond the molecules that make up the matter of the body, we see fields of energy. Ancient Vedic knowledge tells us that this vital energy moves in discretely defined channels, and there exist concentrations of energy in the midline of the body. These centers, or wheels of energy, are called chakras, and each of these centers resonates with a core human need.

When a center is open, the energy that flows through that chakra allows the associated need to be met more effortlessly. When a chakra is blocked, its energy becomes stagnant and intentions are more difficult to actualize. Essential oils are key to keeping these wheels of energy open and flowing smoothly. We can use their vibrational energy to fine-tune our chakral system, bringing the gift aspects of each center forward and shifting the shadow aspects into their positive state.

Chakras: Profiles

The Tattwic Elements are so chthonic, i.e., underground and primal, that the Collective Unconscious of the human race responds to the essence of each element's shape and color. The result is an immediate stirring of the associated chakra.

DR. JOHN MUMFORD,
MAGICAL TATTWAS

The tattva are so intimately connected to the chakras that we must understand the dynamic link that exists between the two. As Dr. Mumford reminds us, to stimulate a tattva is to stir the associated chakra (for example, to stimulate the earth element is to stimulate the root chakra). Following are basic energetic profiles for the seven main chakras. When exploring the chakras, read the profile of the associated tattva first (see chapter 3). The tattva is a denser, primal vibration that is the heart of the evolving energy expressed in a more complex pattern at each chakra.

THE ROOT CHAKRA

All things must come to the soul from its roots, from where it is planted.

SAINT TERESA OF AVILA

Sanskrit Name: Muladhara

Number: First

Location: Base of the spine/coccyx

Tattva Correlation: Earth

Color: Blood red/crimson

Gifts

+ Being grounded, earth connection
+ Stability, security, a sense of belonging
+ Raw sexuality, body pleasure
+ Body knowledge, instinctual knowing
+ Inner security and foundation of self
+ Wise use of earth gifts (i.e., essential oils, crystals, metals/minerals, plant essences)

Shadow Issues

+ Energetically anemic, feeling cut off and isolated
+ Ambivalence toward life, poverty consciousness, substance abuse, or any type of drastic escapism
+ Sex for any type of exchange or just to "feel"
+ Not living in a sustainable way that supports the Earth

THE SACRAL CHAKRA

My soul is screaming in ecstasy.

Rumi

Sanskrit Name: Svadhishthana

Number: Second

Location: Sacrum/pelvic bowl

Tattva Correlation: Water

Color: Vibrant orange

Gifts

+ Sensuality, sexual intimacy, giving and receiving pleasure
+ Creativity, unstructured expression
+ Movement, things that wax and wane
+ Healthy emotions and inner child
+ "Hidden treasure" aspects of self and fluidity
+ Working with dreams and the unconscious

Shadow Issues

+ Wounded emotions, keeping secrets
+ Fear of judgment, "getting in trouble," or "being found out"
+ Repression of aspects of the self, inability to experience emotional or sexual intimacy, manipulation
+ Nightmares or not being able to remember or interpret dreams

THE SOLAR PLEXUS CHAKRA

He is able who thinks he is able.

BUDDHA

Sanskrit Name: Manipura

Number: Third

Location: Solar plexus

Tattva Correlation: Fire

Color: Radiant yellow

Gifts

+ Personal power, the intellect, opinion

+ Logic, will, direction, joy, leadership
+ Action, authority, integrity, radiance
+ Courage, self-worth, consciousness, refinement

Shadow Issues

+ Anger, pettiness, rage, hatred
+ Ego issues, abuse of power (i.e., domination, misguided force, using fear to control)
+ Feeling superior, "my way is the only way"
+ Perfectionism, rigidity, violence, feeling weak
+ Having no expression of personal choice

THE HEART CHAKRA

Your vision will become clear only when you look into your heart. Who looks outside, dreams. Who looks inside, awakens.

CARL JUNG

Sanskrit Name: Anahata

Number: Fourth

Location: Center of the breastbone

Tattva Correlation: Air

Color: Radiant green, radiant pink

Gifts

+ All love: unconditional, romantic, veneration for the divine, parent/child, nature/pets, nonattached, universal
+ Fostering forgiveness, resolving conflicts
+ Union with others and self, transforming the common into the divine

+ Experiencing the divine in self and others
+ Grace, surrender, compassion, loyalty
+ Genuine concern for others and the desire to foster what is best for them, not yourself

Shadow Issues

+ Not accepting self, having only conditional love for self and others, rejecting the magic and beauty surrounding self
+ Being controlling or jealous, demonstrating fear-based affection, using "affection" to manipulate, not allowing others to change or grow
+ Feeling vulnerable or rejected, not allowing others in, not exposing the "real self," codependent relationships
+ Being critical and hard to please, having an exaggerated view of people (whether positive or negative)

THE THROAT CHAKRA

If you can imagine it, you can create it. If you can dream it, you can become it.

WILLIAM ARTHUR WARD

Sanskrit Name: Vishuddha

Number: Fifth

Location: Throat

Tattva Correlation: Ether

Color: Radiant blue

Gifts

+ Truth, expression, sound, clarity, "giving voice to"
+ True vocation, self-expression

+ Clarity, wit, improvisation, spontaneity, active engagement with your inner muse
+ Clairaudience, channeling, telepathy, working with subtle energies
+ Understanding the power of words and how they shape and mold our reality

Shadow Issues

+ Using words or sound irresponsibly
+ Not being an active listener, wordiness, and "speaking at" someone for conversation
+ Not able to discern truth; feeling muddled and confused
+ Disengaged from your inner muse and authentic expression

THE THIRD EYE

It's not what you look at that matters, it's what you see.

HENRY DAVID THOREAU

Sanskrit Name: Ajna

Number: Sixth

Location: Center of the forehead (third eye)

Tattva Correlation: All of the elements combined

Color: Luminescent indigo

Gifts

+ Cosmic knowledge, control of the mind
+ Seeing beyond duality; Shiva's eye (seeing the past, present, future)
+ Sat-chit-ananda: consciousness-being-bliss, embodying all the elements in their purest form; perfect concentration
+ There is no observed or observer: "That I am; I am That."

THE CROWN CHAKRA

Enlightenment is the key to everything.

MARIANNE WILLIAMSON

Sanskrit Name: Sahasrara

Number: Seventh

Location: Crown of the head

Tattva Correlation: Beyond the elements

Color: Luminescent violet or white

Gifts

+ The pure void: no activity of the mind, no knower, nothing to be known, all dissolved into their primary cause
+ Sat-chit-ananda: truth-being-bliss, the highest state of existence
+ The illusion of individual self dissolves, and you are your own real self; enlightenment

5
Emptiness

Releasing Consciousness from Matter

Physical purity alone cannot carry the aspirant to higher dimensions because it is related only to the gross body. Beyond the gross body there are several other bodies or planes of existence related to the hidden layers of the mind.

These are subjected to the influence of samskaras *(latent impressions) which create* sankalpa *and* vikalpa *(thought/counterthought) in the level of the conscious mind. Any disharmony on those levels is immediately transferred to the respective bodies. Just as a physical disease arises out of neglect and carelessness towards the body, there are subtle and causal "diseases" that build up in the* sukshma sharira *(subtle body) and* karana sharira *(causal body) through carelessness in the way we feel, think, react and interact with life.*

SWAMI SATYASANGANANDA

A larger picture of the complex nature of matter is starting to emerge. The common theme in all alchemical-based traditions, including the method we are exploring, is that *the goal is to release consciousness from matter* or to unbind our awareness from the fetters of projection. To

69

release our "inner knowing," we must purify the obstructing overlay of calcified energy. This undertaking, called tattva shuddhi, is a process of purification of the subtle elements that ultimately facilitates moving beyond our own limited awareness and aids in the process of accessing the deepest layers of composted energy from which we are built.

Although we have a great deal of freedom in personal choice and can mindfully engage with each new layer of understanding as it unfurls, dealing with energies we cannot consciously name often confounds us. How do we recognize existing energy patterns and identify the ways in which they influence our life?

In her fascinating essay "An Absurdist Pantomime," psychotherapist Barbara Shore examines the way in which our thought processes shape the data that constitute our perceived reality, including our self and our surroundings.

> We have to make room for the possibility that our thought processes do not neutrally report on what is "out there" in an "objective" world. But rather, like the suppositions of theoretical physicist David Bohm, that our thought processes actively participate in forming our perceptions, our sense of meaning, our daily actions. Bohm suggests that "collective thought and knowledge have become so automated that we're in large part controlled by them, with a subsequent loss of authenticity, freedom and order." Seen through his hypothesis, thought is not a fresh, direct perception but rather is the past—that which has already been thought—carried forward through memory into the present.[1]

In other words, we are hardwired to live in a repeating loop. Our present reality is in large part defined by repeating calcified energy patterns that greatly limit what our awareness can perceive and absorb. Generally speaking, we can only know that which already exists within our realm of awareness, and we must use this small opening of awareness to scan the vast oceans of knowledge and information to begin the process of becoming more aware. I believe that most creation stories are metaphors for this very process of becoming awake or aware—that is, enlightened.

The following section, a discussion of the nature of reality, is quite dense but worth reading again and again. I suggest approaching the information in the same way you would a complicated Tibetan Buddhist teaching: the lama will often read the text, just once, without further explanation, and return to it at a later time. The belief is that the first step in "learning" something new, something that is outside your calcified patterns of perception, is imprinting the information into your continuum and allowing it to ripen, until it flowers in the mind and you are ready to study the new concept in earnest. Read this next section with the energy of positive anticipation that one day soon this concept will ripen in your continuum and become your reality.

Perception and Reality

Author Michael Talbot, who explored the links between ancient philosophy and quantum theory, gives a beautiful explanation concerning ether (the void), the womb of everything, which we cannot perceive with our senses, and the nonvoid, which we experience through our sense organs.

> The Tibetan Buddhists call these two aspects the void and nonvoid. The nonvoid is the reality of visible objects. The void, like implicate order, is the birthplace of all things in the universe, which pour out of it in a "boundless flux." However, only the void is real and all forms in the objective world are illusory, existing merely because of the unceasing flux between the two orders.
>
> In turn, the void is described as "subtle," "indivisible," and "free from distinguishing characteristics." Because it is seamless totality it cannot be described in words. Properly speaking, even the nonvoid cannot be described in words because it, too, is a totality in

which consciousness and matter and all other things are indissoluble and whole. Herein lies a paradox, for despite its illusory nature the nonvoid still contains "an infinitely vast complex of universes." And yet its indivisible aspects are always present. As Tibet scholar John Bloomfield states, "In a universe thus composed, everything interpenetrates, and is interpenetrated by, everything else; as with the void, so with the nonvoid—the part *is* the whole."

The Tibetans prefigured some of [theoretical quantum physicist] Pribram's [theories] as well. According to Milarepa, an eleventh-century Tibetan yogi and the most renowned of the Tibetan Buddhist saints, the reason we are unable to perceive the void directly is because our unconscious mind (or, as Milarepa puts it, our "inner-consciousness") is far too "conditioned" in its perceptions. This conditioning not only keeps us from seeing what he calls "the border between mind and matter," or what we would call the frequency domain, but also causes us to form a body for ourselves when we are in the between-life state and no longer have a body. "In the invisible realm of the heavens . . . the illusory mind is the great culprit," writes Milarepa, who counseled his disciples to practice "perfect seeing and contemplation" in order to realize this "Ultimate Reality."[2]

I want to draw special attention to the statement "The reason we are unable to perceive the void directly is because our unconscious mind . . . is far too 'conditioned' in its perceptions." At this time in our current cultural collective, many fields, from Jungian depth psychology to theoretical physics, seem to be arriving at this idea, which sages from many traditions have brought forward through human existence. Not only are most of us unable to view the void, but most of us are not able to experience even the nonvoid with lucidity!

To break down the calcified patterns that maintain our "conditioned perceptions" (i.e., that which determines how we project our "reality"), we must begin by understanding the nature of matter and how it mediates our present gross reality (i.e., the world we project), and even how it creates the pattern (or self) that we will actualize in our next life. The projection of the gross, or "illusory," mind causes us to reorganize into the form we will take in our next life, for better, for worse, or not at all. (If you do not believe in reincarnation, your karmic projection will still create the afterlife you believe in and project you forward.)

This understanding is also the key that allows us to see which vibrational remedies would best serve our personal evolution, whether that is a specific energetic pattern that needs harmonizing or one that we must develop for next-stage expansion. Clarity surrounding the nature of matter allows us to begin the journey of piercing the veil of illusion (so that we can ultimately experience the void firsthand) and to be truly conscious of the energy that is present and at work in our life (to escape the repeating loop that makes up our collective pattern and to let in fresh energy).

Talbot offers further insight into Bohm's and Pribram's ideas concerning the nature of reality and our quest to understand why human beings organize according to a collective way of perception.

Our brains mathematically construct object reality by interpreting frequencies that are ultimately projection from another dimension, a deeper order of existence that is beyond both space and time: The brain is a hologram enfolded in a holographic universe.*. . . The objective world does not exist, at least not in the way we are accustomed to believing. What is "out there" is a vast ocean of waves and frequencies, and reality looks concrete to us only because our brains are able to take this holographic blur and convert it into the sticks and stones and other familiar objects that make up our world. How is the brain (which itself is composed of frequencies of matter) able to take something as insubstantial as a blur of frequencies and make it seem solid to the touch? . . . The smoothness of a piece of

---

*This is what Deepak Chopra refers to as nonlocal consciousness.

fine china and the feel of beach sand beneath our feet are really just elaborate versions of the phantom limb syndrome. . . . This does not mean there aren't china cups and grains of beach sand out there. It simply means that a china cup has two very different aspects to its reality. When it is filtered through the lens of our brain it manifests as a cup. But if we could get rid of our lenses, we'd experience it as an interference pattern. Which one is real and which is illusion?[3]

When Pribram was posed a question concerning the void/nonvoid and which one is real, he answered, "Both are real to me . . . or, if you want to say, neither of them are real."[4]

This concept is similar to that discussed in the Heart Sutra. When the venerable Shariputra asked Avalokiteshvara, the Buddha of compassion, how to perform the profound activity of perfecting wisdom, he answered:

[One] should clearly see that the five aggregates are also empty of any inherent nature. . . . Similarly, feelings, discriminations, compositional factors, and consciousness are also empty. Likewise, Shariputra, all phenomena are empty. They have no defining characteristics; they are unproduced; they do not cease; they are unstained; they are not separate from stains. They do not decrease nor do they increase.[5]

In the context of the axiom "As above, so below," the nature of existence reveals our connection to all energy and information in the cosmos and clarifies why the Buddhist concept of dependent arising, or creating our own karma or reality, involves so much more than setting intentions or wishful thinking. Becoming clear on what we would like to manifest and holding a correct mental space for it is the first step; next, our physical actions must constantly support the paradigm we want to birth, in conjunction with the proper vibrational tools. Our power to create our reality is illuminated in one of the earliest alchemical texts, the Codex Marcianus. In "The Prophetess Isis to Her Son," one of the pieces of the codex, Isis says:

> Having part of the divine power and being happy about its divine presence, I will now also answer their questions about sands, which one does not prepare from other substances, for one must stay with existing nature and the matter one has in hand in order to prepare things. Just as I said before, wheat creates wheat, and a man begets a man, and thus also gold will harvest gold, like produces like. Now I have manifested the mystery to you.[6]

Here Isis reveals one of the most profound energetic secrets available to humankind: like begets like. Said another way, our actions, thoughts, and use of energetic medicine have formed causation paths that created our present realities and can indeed form our future realities as well. We cannot plant a turnip and expect to grow a tulip. We must plant energetically what we want to produce in our life—gold will harvest gold, wheat creates wheat. We frequently "wake up" to an undesired reality formed from actions laid down long ago (including past-life actions of which we have no mental awareness). Then we must untangle the knot of energy, combing and smoothing it out, until we can start the process of weaving the next chapter of our life.

In *How Karma Works,* Geshe Sonam Rinchen explains causation with a similar metaphor.

> The sunflower seed is an impermanent condition because it itself came into existence through other causes and conditions. At the moment when it ceases, its result, the sunflower seedling, appears. The sunflower seed is a condition with potential because it has the specific capacity to produce a sunflower—something that is related to it—and will not produce any other kind of flower. The presence of a healthy sunflower seed and the other essential conditions will produce a sunflower. It will not come into existence without the

presence of that seed nor will a zinnia seed produce a sunflower. So the sunflower does not come into being causelessly nor from discordant causes.[7]

Each of us holds remarkable potential for conscious creation and the ability to be present. The work of freeing our soul from the fetters of the body (matter) to gain sight beyond naive projection molds not only how we perceive our environment but also how we project our understanding of self and others in our lives. This act depends on understanding the play between matter and energy and how this creates our reality.

PART 2

Essential Oils

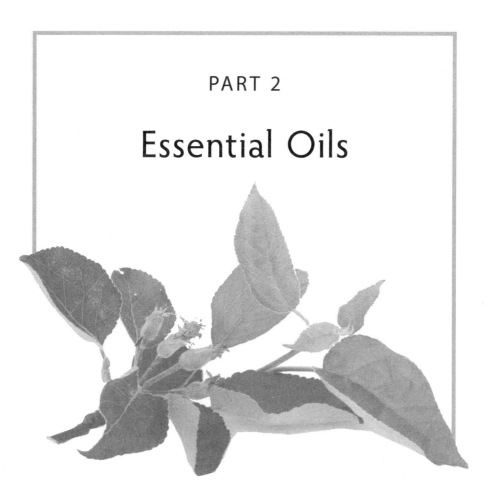

6

Essential Oils
for Spiritual Alchemy

There are many dimensions to every plant. One of the most beautiful celebrations of the complex range of healing that plants offer comes from the *Rig Veda,* in which a doctor petitions the plants for help: "Mothers, you have a hundred forms and a thousand growths. You who have a hundred ways of working, make this man whole for me."

The profiles of essential oils in this chapter cannot possibly cover the breadth of each plant's energy and effects, but the information provided will get you started. (I encourage you to delve independently into each oil's healing secrets.) When reading the descriptions, *take all of the information into account* to understand how the essential oils will operate in your energetic body. Know that the use of an essential oil to stimulate a tattva has the following implications: awakening the archetypal associations in your being; striking the resonant chord within you that corresponds to the elemental arrangements; and stimulating the corresponding chakra. Read with an open mind and heart, and find the micro- and macrocosm within yourself that elegantly connects you with all of creation.

Essential Oil Bottling Considerations

Essential oils should be stored in glass bottles that support your intent. The most common type used are simply dark glass bottles as these protect the chemical constituents of essential oils—although when bottling for energetics you have more leeway. For example, you may choose to use a special green glass bottle when working with the heart chakra or air element, as this color will support your overall intent. I even use frosted white glass bottles as they impart uplifting and purifying energy. If you use common sense and keep your bottles out of direct sunlight all colors are suitable.

Violet glass, which appears more black than violet, is fascinating because only infrared, violet, and ultraviolet light can pass through it, as opposed to the "rainbow spectrum" we can see with our naked eye. Violet glass protects the vibrational aspect of the essential oil, preserving its archetypal morphic field. For example, let's assume that you are in crisis due to a circumstance in your life and you have acquired an essential oil to assist in healing the crisis. The energy from which you seek to escape is pervasive in your environment; this energy would affect everything in the area, including any essential oils you have. As we have discussed, liquid is one of the best templates on which to inscribe vibrational information. While it is marvelous to have such a dynamic means to distribute subtle information, there has always been a problem with keeping the vibrational integrity of products pure.

The color spectrum governs different bodies of knowledge, as follows:

- Infrared governs **instinct:** body knowing and instinctual perceptions.
- Rainbow colors govern **personal or experiential knowledge:** personal karma and causality from life.
- Ultraviolet governs **archetypes:** information from the unconscious, information from Source, and dream images.

A violet glass bottle allows the information contained within the instinctual and archetypal energy fields of the plants being used to interact freely with the contents of the bottle, enlivening the liquid and keeping it vital and potent, without distortion, while keeping the "emotion-based" energy of the rainbow color spectrum at bay. This is not to say that the color spectrum of the plant is not active but rather that the contents are not manipulated by external factors that resonate with human imbalance.

Working with the subtle bodies is different from working with the physical body. We do not rely on the chemical compounds found within essential oils to be the catalyst for movement. Instead, we are connecting with the complex, subtle information that is archetypically expressed within the morphic field of each plant/essential oil, which forms the architecture that allows us to literally alter the shape of our energetic body.

Remember that one type of bottle is not universally better than another. Each provides a specific vibration that may be appropriate depending on your current needs. Myself, I use violet glass for my tattvas oils, frosted glass for my chakra blends, and amber glass for my Ganesha blend. what is "done" w/them?

Essential Oils
to Stimulate the Tattvas

The five essential oils that I use to stimulate the tattvas are energetic adaptogens, meaning that they create balance in the energetic field. When you incorporate them into your personal practice, know that what needs to be brought forward will be (the gift aspects), and what needs to be healed will be as well (balancing the shadow aspects). If a certain aspect of an essential oil's energetic profile resonates with you, it is beneficial to work with that aspect with focused intent.

The tattva essential oils provide a range of benefits, such as the following:

+ They actively engage the mental body as we intellectually explore the plant and its archetypal and elemental actions. This allows us to consciously engage with the healing vibrations in our practice.

✦ They vibrationally impart information that addresses the whole of the self and engages with the deep self, before the conscious aspect of self is able to grasp the knowledge. This is akin to tilling and preparing the soil—from the deep, fecund, unconscious aspects of self, the vibrations stimulate the germination that allows conscious understanding to come fully into awareness.

✦ With their strong fragrance and volatile constituents, they have a unique connection to the limbic brain and thus deal dynamically with the instinctual aspect of self. This includes the "irrational" soul and the emotional aspects of a human being that make being human so confusing at times. Essential oils are uniquely qualified to work with the "repository of self," or karmic birth patterns—traits that are so deeply ingrained that they feel solid and immutable.

The fragrance of an essential oil reinforces the information imparted vibrationally, intellectually, and visually. For example, betel leaf essential oil's scent has a distinctly smoky base note. It first hits the nose as dark, woodsy, mossy, moist, vegetal, and acrid, followed by a dry-out note that smells of spring—the scent of rainfall, with a slightly sweet floral note. The smoky base note speaks to radical form shift, as fire produces smoke and is one of the quickest and most dynamic ways to free matter from its present form. The seed of ether speaks to matter's endless possibilities for reformatting before taking form and entering rebirth, which is fragrantly portrayed here as spring. The fragrance "paints" the same death/rebirth story that the elements, colors, archetypal pattern, and plant express.

AGARWOOD
(*Gahuaru buaya*)

Element: Ether, with seed of water

Catalyst for: Introspection, revelation, deep wisdom

Chakra Correlation: Fifth (vishuddha, throat), second (svadhishthana, pelvic bowl)

Sacred Syllables: *Ham, vam*

Key Vibrations:
Gifts: helps you gain an understanding of and access to the akashic field (ether); aids the mind in perceiving circumstance and environment as a gestalt; promotes open-mindedness and positive boundaries.

Balancing: helps you take inventory of your personal reality, with the intent to understand your emotions (water) and how they may be detracting from your full involvement with life; removes layers of reflexive emotional states to aid you in being able to be present in whatever is authentically occurring in the moment.

Key Concepts: The combination of ether and water gives rise to the energy of *daring*. This is an expansive combination that promotes reaching new heights on all levels. This process begins by looking inward. Ether is boundless space, holding all possibilities, while water, seeping ever downward, connects to and purifies the unconscious and emotional aspects of self, seeking the lowest ground to be contained (paradoxically, the "container" is boundless space or endless expansion). Are there any contracted, distorted, or unexpressed aspects of self that need to be explored, purified, and allowed to blossom?

From this inward exploration, you can move outward. Agarwood provides the framework for moving outside of your comfort zone, allowing for dynamic new growth. This may mean achieving new levels of personal success, finding emotional freedom, or loosening your current bonds and soaring to new spiritual heights.

Deity Archetype: Sarasvati, goddess of wisdom
Agarwood essential oil vibrates to a bright emanation of the divine feminine in the form of Sarasvati, goddess of wisdom. This archetypal expression relates to the plant's elemental arrangement of ether with the

seed of water. Priya Hemenway writes that Sarasvati "is a water deity and is symbolic of the pool of knowledge that runs parallel to creation. In the form of a river she runs from the mountains to the sea, moving through and nourishing all the realms of human existence."[1]

In addition to being the goddess of wisdom, Sarasvati is also a virginal goddess in the original context of the term, meaning "unto one's self." She never had children and did not favor being married—in fact, she got the boot from Brahma because she could never rally behind the idea of being a "good wife." Instead, she devoted her time to the acquisition of knowledge and the development of self and the arts, including speech and the written word (skills that facilitate sharing the wisdom and insight you acquire).

Agarwood's primary element is ether, which carries the vibration of sound, expression, and the gift of speech, which are believed to be the very source of creation. This aspect of agarwood amplifies your work with mantras (sacred syllables) and the ability to use speech mindfully to create your reality.

These qualities make agarwood an excellent choice for determining which path is worthwhile and ushering in, calibrating, and crystallizing new vibrational patterns—an incredible combination.

Incantation: Sarasvati, uttering your very name helps transform mere knowledge into spiritual truth. I appeal to you to facilitate the expansion of my knowledge into wisdom. Support my desire that my heart, mind, and actions always reflect this wisdom and that I understand and become one with universal truth.

Animal Archetype: White Heron

This archetype carries the energy of self-reflection. Other traits include active patience, determination, innovation, self-reliance, balance, self-evolution, independence, intelligence, strength, the wisdom of considering all options, thinking outside the box, and expressing uniqueness.

Suggestions for Practical Use: Use agarwood to amplify communication, effective listening skills, and expression. Use it to purify inharmonious emotional states, to gain access to timeless wisdom, and for support in artistic expression (music, painting, writing, etc.). Use it in mantra, prayer, and meditation practices. It supports being whole unto one's self.

Note: Agarwood sometimes comes in the form of a resin that needs to be liquefied before use; simply bring a small saucepan of water to a boil, reduce the heat to low, and set the agarwood bottle in the hot water. Let the bottle sit in the hot water until its contents become liquid.

BETEL LEAF
(Piper betle)

Element: Fire, with seed of ether

Catalyst for: Balancing the ego, radical form shift, and releasing consciousness from matter

Chakra Correlation: Third (manipura, solar plexus), fifth (vishuddha, throat)

Sacred Syllables: *Ram, ham*

Key Vibrations:
Gifts: enriches understanding through cycles; transmutes disturbances on the mental, physical, spiritual, or emotional level; allows rebirth into a new form—one more in accord with what has been learned through the most recent expression of self; aids in releasing consciousness from matter; allows information stored at a cellular and energetic level to be made known to the conscious mind for use.

Balancing: addresses fear surrounding deep behavioral changes and changes in external reality; helps you overcome a being disconnected from instinctual wisdom and body knowledge.

Key Concepts: The combination of fire and ether gives rise to the energy of *transmutation*. This is the process of understanding the root of unwholesome energy and changing that energy's form from its limiting state into its beneficial state.

Deity Archetype: The Dark Goddess in her undifferentiated form

I believe that the energetic taproot of all of the Dark Goddess's manifestations is the dark moon. These manifestations include, but are not limited to, Lilith, Palden Lhamo, Black Tara, Hecate, and the Black Madonna. In her book *Mysteries of the Dark Moon: The Healing Power of the Dark Goddess,* Demetra George provides a beautiful exposition on the dark moon. I love her descriptions of the eight lunation phases, particularly what she calls the Depth of Dark and the Dark Dawning, the phases immediately preceding and following the dark moon.

Depth of Dark

At the Balsamic Phase, the life impulse distills and concentrates the wisdom of the entire cycle into a capsule of seed ideas for future visions. During the dark of the moon, the life force transforms the past into a mutation of the future and makes a commitment to seeding new concepts within old structures. The symbolic seed once again turns back into itself.

Dark Dawning

At the New Phase, the flow of solar-lunar energy emerges, initiates and projects the seed impulse in an instinctive and subjective manner that will fulfill and complete a purpose as the remaining cycle unfolds. In the absence of light, the vision is felt, not seen. The symbolic seed germinates underground.[2]

From an elemental perspective, the Depth of Dark phase corresponds to the element ether (the dark/dry void), which rips asunder, helping to pull apart, dissolve, and undo outmoded patterns of behavior, and offers the distilled and concentrated wisdom of the previous cycle. This occurs in the darkness, in our unconscious mind. The Dark

Dawning phase corresponds to the element fire, which acts as a shunt from the unconscious to the conscious, allowing us to harvest that which was sown in the darkness.

Incantation: Mother, divine, black, and perfect, I call upon you to rip asunder all that is incorrect, to give me the strength to hold my position against all opposition, and to call to me all who will support my journey into wholeness as I birth my new way of being. Hold me in the velvet of your arms. Feed me and cradle me as I grow out of your dark perfection. Amen.

Animal Archetype: Snake

Snake brings authentic growth, growth through cycles, using potions to heal, the Dark Goddess, deep magic, alchemy, transmutation, kundalini (serpent's power), and shakti. Snake's energy is that of ancient wisdom and the dynamic experience of radical awakening and shifts in awareness.

Suggestions for Practical Use: Use betel leaf for releasing information "stored within" and using this information for dynamic action in the material world; for facilitating the flow of information from the unconscious to the conscious; and for sparking epiphanies. Use it for stress headaches related to overthinking; for support when you are going through internal or external change; for issues dealing with the ego, whether it is overinflated or diminished; and to help create balance in your life.

GALANGAL
(*Alpinia galanga*)

Element: Earth, with seed of water

Catalyst for: Seeing synchronicities and benefiting from them

Chakra Correlation: First (muladhara, coccyx), second (svadhishthana, pelvic bowl)

Sacred Syllables: *Lam, vam*

Key Vibrations:

Gifts: helps you with understanding that the body is the present focus of personal consciousness and that cosmic consciousness is not "out there" but resonating within you; with being sacramentally rooted in self and surroundings; with knowing that your environment is alive and reacts to your awareness; with being the commander of your own form and reality; with taking pleasure in being alive.

Balancing: helps you with achieving the awareness that life does not happen to you; with ending internal isolation by merging with the divine; with bringing goals to fruition through focused attention and activity, leading to abundance.

Key Concepts: The combination of earth and water gives rise to the energy of *fertility*. This is a nurturing combination that promotes boldness in following your ambitions. Earth provides the firm foundation in which to plant ideas, while water nourishes ideas to fruition, ultimately allowing a harvest.

Deity Archetype: Lakshmi, goddess of fortune

Lakshmi is the Hindu goddess of wealth, prosperity, and generosity and the embodiment of beauty, grace, and charm. She is associated with the lotus and also known by the names Padma, "lotus," and Karisin, "rich in dung." Her names reveal the rich energy she offers. The lotus teaches that you must pass through stages of development and growth to reach the sweet-smelling full bloom of self. The lotus starts its life humbly, in the muck below the waterline, and reaches faithfully upward toward the sun until it attains its full expression of beauty. The name Karisin speaks to the fruit that can be harvested from the labor of wise action. No matter which name Lakshmi presents under, her gift is the same—one of achieving goals and fulfilling your full potential gracefully, thereby opening the way to prosperity through talent, steady work, and a little luck.

Incantation: Lakshmi, your grace is like the full-blooming lotus. Please endow me with your attributes and blessings. Shower wealth into my life, and bring this light by the ripening of my talents and understanding of the correct expression of my gifts. Please open the lotus in my heart and take away the darkness of self-doubt, stagnation, fear, and procrastination. Allow every breath I take to be one of grace, enabling me to move forward in beautiful expression.

Animal Archetype: Otter

The elements of earth and water are primordial feminine energy (but remember that both men and women house this energy). Otter is at home in both of these elements and is an expression of the divine feminine in her bright manifestation. She holds the energy of being playful, creative, exploratory, joyful, beautiful, and grace filled. She not only celebrates her own good fortune but also the unique talents of others. Because Otter is not competitive or jealous, she is open to the many opportunities life offers her. She is the "way bringer," and because she allows events to unfold naturally through the flow of divine support, she is always where she needs to be at exactly the right moment.

Suggestions for Practical Use: Use galangal to support you in taking projects to fruition, for aid in the development of talent, and for bringing you into alignment with beneficial circumstances. This essential oil supports noncompetitive exchange, self-love, and love for being in your body, and it nurtures grace of spirit (social graces) and movement (good for dancers, etc.).

KAFFIR LIME LEAF
(Citrus hystrix)

This oil may be photosensitizing (it may cause hypersensitivity to the sun). Therefore, it is not recommended for topical full-body application less than twenty-four hours prior to full sun exposure.

Element: Air, with seed of fire

Catalyst for: Energetic protection and energetic cord cutting; supports liberation from limiting thoughts and behavioral patterns

Chakra Correlation: Fourth (anahata, heart), third (manipura, solar plexus)

Sacred Syllables: *Yam, ram*

Key Vibrations:

Gifts: helps you to become technique oriented and to delight in the details of working toward practical ends; gives rise to the energy of the specialist, which allows you to establish order and transform your environment by formulating your findings in a technical manner; allows you to determine which tool would be best used in a certain environment.

Balancing: allows you to take information/data and create a repeatable process; aids in understanding the environment of self.

Key Concepts: The combination of air and fire gives rise to the energy of *beneficial combinations.* Air and fire support each other: fire needs air to survive and thrive, and air enjoys giving itself to support fire's dance. This dynamic promotes the energy of positive exchange—joyful giving and receiving—and mutual support. This combination encourages the release of any energetic exchange that is not wholesome and mutually supportive. Consequently, kaffir lime leaf supports exchanges of self in group dynamics, facilitating your own personal growth as well as the growth of others.

Deity Archetype: Green and Red Tara

Tara, a fully enlightened Buddha, has twenty-one classic emanations. If you are not sure which Tara you need, you can call on "all into one," or Green Tara. Green Tara *is* the enlightened air element. Invoking her is the purest expression of air, which rules higher love and compassion. She swiftly removes all hindrances from your temporal path and expands your capacity for genuine love. Her energy facilitates compassionate action in the material world, even when it seems impossible to achieve all you need. You see her energy in mythic individuals like Mother Teresa and in hardworking heroes who ask for no recognition, like Jane Coyle of the Vietnam Fund for Education, Music & Infrastructure. Call upon Tara to help *you* work miracles of kindness on Earth.

Red Tara is the Ripener, or Bestower of Maturity. She is ruby red, and her specialties are subduing hindrances, protecting from fear and danger, and drawing in auspicious energy. Red Tara's wisdom fire is unique: it holds the power to *burn the causes of cyclic existence*, karma and unharmonious patterns, which leads to liberation and enlightenment.

Incantation (for compassionate action): Tara, imbue me with the wisdom and strength to be like you, "quick like lightning" in recognizing and aiding others in need, be it hunger of spirit and soul or need on the physical level. Allow me to see the most skillful and swift means of balancing any imbalance. Help me move forward until every one of my brothers' and sisters' needs are met with the same standards I require for myself, be it the need for education, freedom of thought and expression, ample resources, a healthy environment, or a safe, positive space that encourages growth. Bless me with the divine sensitivity not to push my understanding of good but to ask what each individual requires to flourish and honor that as I meet and interact with each new energy.

Animal Archetype: Red Dragonfly

Red Dragonfly signifies the essence of the winds of change; messages of wisdom and enlightenment from the elemental world; stripping away illusions and recognizing the truth behind form; belief in divine providence; allowing self to be cared for and supported by this energy.

Suggestions for Practical Use: Kaffir lime leaf can help you develop specialization in your desired field so as to cultivate mutually beneficial outcomes and clear inharmonious energies. It magnetizes beneficial energies, excellent for positive group dynamics and organizing your thoughts and environment (yes, this does include cleaning out your closet!), and supports altruistic work, fund-raising, and working for causes.

MASSOIA BARK
(*Cryptocarya massoia*)

This oil may be sensitizing. If used as a topical oil, perform a skin patch test before use, and always use a high dilution rate. For application to the body, I recommend starting with 1 to 3 drops of essential oil for every 3 tablespoons of base oil, seeing how your body reacts, and adjusting from there. If you have any reaction at all, stop topical application and use as a diffusion or for ritual anointing. Never use in the bath.

Element: Earth, with seed of water and seed of air

Catalyst for: Peeling back the layers of the false self

Chakra Correlation: First (muladhara, coccyx), second (svadhishthana, pelvic bowl), fourth (anahata, heart)

Sacred Syllables: *Lam, vam, yam*

Key Vibrations:
Gifts: helps you understand symbols and the complex nature and layers of information they contain (this includes but is not limited to what Hindu philosophers refer to as *maya,* loosely translated as "illusion," which addresses projections—collective and individual).

Balancing: allows you to interpret the rich symbolism that makes your life, including dream imagery; helps you identify projections around yourself so that you can better understand the quality of human togetherness at any particular time and place; helps you determine your own individual stage of evolution.

Key Concepts: The combination of earth (body), water (emotions/soul), and air (mind/spirit) gives rise to the energy of *structured dynamism.*

This energy can be understood as an open-ended and transformative quest that favors unregulated organization through spontaneous order, understanding that true response can only occur in the moment, when all the latent energy of available aspects comes together, allowing a specific dynamic to occur. This concept does not favor a philosophy of stasis with the intent of maintaining the status quo but instead promotes response and adaptation to needs and actions authentically rising in the moment.

Earth is the sacred vessel, or container, in which spontaneous order may arise, allowing the air and water elements to express new combinations of personal divinity as the need develops, in a safe and grounded way.

Deity Archetype: Mother of Creation

This is a fascinatingly complex archetype. She is literally the beginning, the beauty in between, and the end. She is the undivided primal waters, the individual expression of this energy, and the energy that ends and reabsorbs its expression for rebirth. In her wrathful form, she provides the means and the way to slay the ego with divine knowledge to attain *moksha* (liberation, release). She is known by the names Kore, Demeter, Persephone, Raja Rajewari, Durga, Kali, Uma, and the Venus of Willendorf, to name a few. Each of these emanations gives rise to a specific set of actions that teach an aspect of feminine growth, be it the innocent child, sexual adult, mother, destroyer, or crone.

Most schools of thought believe that Sanskrit is a language of dynamism (meaning that it possesses great energy or force), and many Hindu schools believe that each of the letters represents a form of energy, or a form of the Mother of Creation. Therefore, she is generally seen as the mother of language in her aspect of Kali or Sarasvati. She is pure consciousness and has no permanent qualities. Rather, she emanates in whatever form of the divine feminine is required to stretch, reform, and teach the devotee to achieve an intended expansion. Dualistic concepts and rigid forms do not apply to her—she is pure, unmanifested energy. This perspective speaks to the concept of structured dynamism: the exploration of what spontaneous combination of self needs to arise at any given time.

Incantation: Mother of Creation, you are the root source of life, the undivided primal waters, and the place from which all potential rises. Please help me understand that a multitude of expressions are required in this life and grant me the ability to spontaneously adapt to each moment. Remind me that this is not a false way of being but rather truth, as it is against nature to be immutable. Allow me the flexibility of soul to experience all of creation through my being.

Animal Archetype: Loon

Loon is an expression of energy that helps you go the distance into the discovery of true self—to dive deep into your subconscious, emotions, and the collective unconscious and find the gifts that await you. Loon helps you understand your dreams, which are a powerful means of communication with your deep self and the collective unconscious. This energy also helps you separate the real from the unreal, but ultimately it teaches you the powerful gift of active imagination, visualization, and becoming the active dreamer instead of the dreamed. As Loon's name reflects, it takes a bit of "madness" to let go of convention and allow an authentic expression of the ever-evolving self in the moment. This mysterious bird nests on earth, finds sustenance in water, and takes to the air in flight.

Suggestions for Practical Use: Massoia bark essential oil can aid you in spontaneously adapting to new situations and reorganizing yourself and your environment as needed. Use it for powerful, vivid dream work (many users of this oil have noted this effect) and for assistance in "unsticking" from cloying experiences that do not feel like they have been self-generated but seem to ensnare you.

Caution: It is critical to perform a skin patch test of massoia bark essential oil before use. In some people, the sesquiterpene lactones in massoia bark can cause contact dermatitis, often with serious complications, such as inflammation of the skin, possibly over the entire body, and shortness of breath. Though massoia bark does carry some risk, temper your caution with common sense. As chemist and aromatherapist Kurt Schnaubelt, Ph.D., notes, with regard to essential oils with a high potential to cause sensitization, "to entirely take these oils out of circulation or to advise a user to avoid them completely is equivalent to throwing the baby out with the bathwater."[3]

I must stress the importance of using correct dosages. While my healing method system is not focused on the physical body, every essential oil has active chemical compounds that do affect the physical body and must be treated with respect. Less is always more. Please see the "Dosages and Dilutions" section (page 109) for instructions on how to perform a proper skin patch test and proper dilution rates.

Essential Oils to Stimulate the Chakras

There are many essential oils that resonate with each chakra. As we discussed earlier in this book, like all of creation the chakras arise from the tattvas, and essential oils that carry the energy of a particular tattva can directly affect the associated chakra. In fact, essential oils that vibrate with the energy of more than one tattva can stimulate more than one chakra. Jasmine is a noteworthy example: This essential oil is often associated with the sexual aspect of nature and its healing power focused on the second chakra. This is true and a very good fit, but equally as true in the Vedic tradition is the fact that this plant, in conjunction with mantras, is dynamic for mind training, so it is a good stimulant for the sixth chakra. Remember as you read these profiles that each plant's vibration is multifaceted. We are focusing here on just a small aspect of each essential oil's healing power. I have found these essential oils to be especially potent for the chakras I've listed with them, and to keep things from getting confusing I will focus on the aspects of each essential oil that directly relate to the chakra listed with it.

BLACK PEPPER
(*Piper nigrum*)

Element: Fire

Stimulates: Third chakra

Key Vibrations: Living your personal code of conduct, precision, being a specialist

The name for this essential oil in Sanskrit is *marich,* meaning "sun." As its name signifies, this oil holds vast amounts of solar energy and illuminates the mental body (ayurveda teaches that the mental body is produced by the third chakra). Black pepper essential oil at the third chakra allows you to release and transform rigid patterns held by the mind, brings the knowledge that you do not have to repeat the past, and lights the way to seeing new solutions to old problems. This oil also brings the gift of refining an idea into its best expression and living in integrity.

BLOOD ORANGE
(*Citrus sinensis*)

Element: Water, with seed of fire

Stimulates: Second and third chakras

Key Vibrations: Emotional warmth, positive inner child, creativity

This warming essential oil brings the gifts of being happy, emotionally regenerated, strongly self-confident, and sympathetic. If you are troubled by depression, apathy, or an obsessive nature, or if you are healing from emotional abuse, this essential oil will support you.

BLUE CHAMOMILE
(*Matricaria chamomilla*)

Element: Ether, with seed of water

Stimulates: Fifth and second chakras

Key Vibrations: Wisdom, communication, expansion

This sagacious oil helps you cultivate a profound knowledge base on any particular topic; it helps you understand ideas from past eras. It supports you in opening up to guidance from your higher self and spiritual guides, stabilizing this connection, and allowing you to communicate your discoveries. It is a very good oil for writers and artisans.

CARDAMOM
(*Elettaria cardamomum*)

Element: Fire, with seed of water

Stimulates: Third and second chakras

Key Vibrations: Feeling encouraged, enthusiastic, and confident

This motivational essential oil stimulates creativity, opening unexplored parts of the psyche that bring new perspective and understanding. It is an incredible oil for dissolving the patterns of being inflexible, judgmental, and contrary; in turn, this shift opens the ability to work in collectives in a joyful manner.

ELEMI
(*Canarium luzonicum*)

Element: Fire, with seed of ether

Stimulates: Third and fifth chakras

Key Vibrations: Elevating, illuminating, changing perspective

This fascinating resin takes its name from an Arabic term meaning "above and below," and, not surprisingly, elemi essential oil is dynamic for connecting the mind and spirit and for supporting an understanding of the microcosm/macrocosm relationship. This in turn allows your own higher guidance to open you to different perspectives on life, supporting you in taking actions that allow true growth. It is also helpful for exploring your experience of self.

FRANKINCENSE
(Boswellia carteri)

Element: Ether

Stimulates: Fifth chakra

Key Vibrations: Inspiration, mysticism, expression

This remarkable essential oil opens the ability to read energy in environments so that you understand how best to react in the moment from an evolved space. This oil also brings the gifts of refinement in speech, helping you to find the right words for yourself and to use words to affect your environment. It also allows you to tap in to your inner muse for authentic self-expression.

JASMINE
(Jasminum grandiflorum)

Element: All of the elements

Stimulates: All of the chakras, but especially the second and sixth

Key Vibrations: Sensitivity, nonordinary senses, refinement

In Vedic thought this oil promotes psychic ability that makes the mind open and insightful. Traditionally this oil has been used for making the mind sensitive to the frequency of mantras, so it can be of benefit for a chanting or prayer practice. It also has a refining quality.

LAVENDER
(*Lavandula officinalis*)

Element: Ether

Stimulates: Fifth chakra

Key Vibrations: Healing, soothing, cushioning

Lavender harmonizes more aspects of the human condition than any other essential oil. This remarkable oil encourages you to deeply engage with the world, sharing your unique gifts and light. This oil heals feelings of being overly delicate, withdrawn, or fearful and brings spiritual growth by helping you integrate your experiences, which brings an expanded awareness and perspective.

LEMON
(*Citrus limon*)

Element: Fire in association with the third chakra; *prabhava** in relation to the sixth chakra

Stimulates: Third chakra; sixth chakra

Key Vibrations in association with the third chakra: Deep purification, versatility, clarity of mind

This electrifying essential oil is very stimulating; it helps organize the mind and brings concentration, boundless energy, and freshness of thought. If you are struggling with mental fatigue that leads to mental blocks and inner turmoil, this essential oil offers relief. It can also be helpful for overcoming feelings of bitterness or hypersensitivity and for the individual who has lost their sense of humor.

---

*This Sanskrit word translates to mean "special quality." Plants (that essential oils are distilled from) occasionally rise above the general schemata for understanding their behavior and have specific qualities that transcend thought, displaying uniqueness beyond any general rules. Lemon falls into this category.

Key vibrations in relation to the sixth chakra: Light, awareness, illumination

This oil has the ability to bathe the pineal gland with light, helping to awaken latent gifts of the third eye. It offers the gift of connecting the mental body to intuition, creating mental versatility and an expanded thought process, while simultaneously helping the mind organize the influx of new information so you do not become overwhelmed with all the new information flowing in.

LIME
(*Citrus aurantifolia*)

Element: Prabhava

Stimulates: Seventh chakra

Key Vibrations: Release, detachment, freedom

This essential oil is beneficial for energetic cord cutting and detaching from the collective. Use it to enhance your perception of the truth inside any situation, which allows you to release any illusion that keeps you ensnared in a projected reality.

NEROLI
(*Citrus aurantium*)

Element: Air, with seed of water

Stimulates: Fourth and second chakras

Key Vibrations: Spirituality, completeness in self, serenity

This refined essential oil is a delight! Bringing the energy of pure love and lightness of being, she melts away sorrows and brings a peaceful, stable calm. This oil is indispensable for healing trauma from childhood abuse or anytime you are in an emotional crisis or suffering from sadness; she fosters a sense of hope and leads you from fear. Neroli also opens you to love within yourself and the freedom of allowing love to flow freely.

PATCHOULI
(*Pogostemon cablin*)

Element: Earth, with seed of water

Stimulates: First and second chakras

Key Vibrations: Unruffled, lucid, gathering personal energy back to self

This self-contained essential oil gives the gift of enjoying being alone with yourself in a content, relaxed state; this in turn gives rise to having a large energy store so you can get things done. It can be very supportive in helping you reach your goals, from clarification of what you desire to having the tenacity to do what is needed to reach fulfillment. This essential oil also helps you overcome fatigue and feeling downhearted.

PINE
(*Pinus sylvestris*)

Element: Air, with seed of fire

Stimulates: Fourth and third chakras

Key Vibrations: Self-love, self-forgiveness, trust

Pine is a key essential oil for restoration of the heart when your emotions have hardened. This loving oil releases you from old wounds, letting you move forward without the baggage of the past, bringing the ability to experience your emotions in real time versus playing out echoes from the past. This shift allows your emotional body to be nourished and replenished, bringing growth, inner peace, a strong sense of well-being, and the ability to engage in loving relationships.

PINK PEPPER SEED
(*Schinus molle*)

Element: Fire, with seed of water

Stimulates: Second and third chakras

Key Vibrations: Inner trust, inner warmth, expressiveness

This spicy essential oil opens your erotic, rapturous nature and love to be in your body. This gives rise to ecstatic sexuality and supports the healing of shame, body image issues, frigidity, and feelings of vulnerability.

RED SPIKENARD
(*Nardostachys jatamansi*)

Element: Prabhava

Stimulates: Balances all of the chakras

Key Vibrations: Grounding of spirituality, body wisdom, access to ancient information

Red spikenard addresses subconscious traumas. It is grounding, but not in a dulling way; it allows you to gain control of your life and help stabilize you when you are feeling unsafe in your physical body. Use this oil to shunt the energy from your upper chakras to your first chakra to ground those energies for practical use. Also beneficial for those on a spiritual path, to balance the mundane with the elevated as in the Zen saying "Before enlightenment, chop wood, carry water. After enlightenment, chop wood, carry water."

CHINESE RICE FLOWER
(*Aglaia odorata*)

Element: Prabhava

Stimulates: Seventh chakra

Key Vibrations: Study, mysteries, thresholds

This profound essential oil is beneficial for contemplating life's great mysteries and acts as a portal between the temporal and the divine. It is supportive when you are reading philosophy or spirituality books, as it helps you understand how to transform ideas into action. One of the more fascinating gifts that this oil imparts is the ability to hold on to an idea that feels too big, too vast—without shutting down or leaving the process—until your mind is finally able to penetrate its mystery.

ROSE
(*Rosa damascena*)

Element: Prabhava

Stimulates: Fourth and seventh chakras

Key Vibrations: Love, grace, enlightenment

Rose essential oil stimulates the desire to work toward enlightenment via the path of the heart. Love being the key to unfolding the path at each stage of development, this is a route filled with grace that teaches strength in gentleness, which results in harmonious actions. It is a very good oil if you do not want to attend the school of hard knocks along the way.

ROSEWOOD
(*Aniba rosaeodora*)

Element: Air

Stimulates: Fourth chakra

Key Vibrations: Protection, cushioning, comfort

This beautiful essential oil encourages free-flowing emotions, the ability to harmonize what you are feeling with your thoughts, and the capacity to express a full range of emotions, especially those related to releasing pain and sadness. This oil offers strong energetic protection and can help you maintain a clean and enclosed aura. Use it for releasing constricted feelings stored in the chest, internalized grief, melancholy, and repressed emotions.

SANDALWOOD
(*Santalum album*)

Element: Prabhava

Stimulates: Sixth chakra

Key Vibrations: Enlightenment, meditation, connection

This wise oil brings an inner awareness and a sense of ease engaging with higher consciousness, which is helpful for insights into blockages on your spiritual path, whether internal or external, and allows a gentle processing at your deepest levels. Ultimately sandalwood helps break down illusions, helping you align with your most authentic self. This is an excellent oil for meditation, spiritual practice, and healers.

VANILLA
(*Vanilla planifolia*)

Element: Water

Stimulates: Second chakra

Key Vibrations: Positive sexuality, commitment, fulfillment

This sweet-smelling essential oil is highly viscous, and its physical form reveals many of its energetic traits. Using this essential oil helps you create emotional bonds and the desire to follow your heart. It gives rise to personal passion, sexuality, wildness, and touch as a form of communication. It helps heal emotional conflicts, oversensitivity, bitterness, hostility, insincerity, and resentment. It gives rise to being unselfish and truly understanding what is required to be in a balanced partnership.

VETIVER
(*Vetiveria zizanioides*)

Element: Earth, with seed of fire

Stimulates: First and third chakras

Key Vibrations: Integrity, protection, serenity

This rich essential oil brings the gifts of being grounded and centered in self. This in turn cultivates the traits of strength, being honorable, and a strong mind-body connection. If you are struggling with loss of purpose and finding the correct direction, this is an excellent essential oil to aid you with finding the right path forward.

WHITE LOTUS
(*Nelumbo nucifera*)

Element: All of the elements

Stimulates: All of the chakras

Key Vibrations: Growth, soul, spirit

White lotus holds the vibration of the entire path of enlightenment and is a powerful teacher and guide. This radiant oil first stimulates you at the unconscious level, bringing the desire to become self-actualized, and then supports this path as your budding consciousness learns the lessons offered from each chakral center. Of course, the ultimate goal of this oil is to usher you in to a state of enlightenment. This is an excellent oil to reach for when you cannot quite name what has you stuck, but you know you need relief, as lotus supports your whole life journey and circumstances.

SUMMARY OF CHAKRA / ESSENTIAL OIL CORRESPONDENCES

CHAKRA	ESSENTIAL OIL
First (muladhara/root)	Galangal, massoia bark, patchouli, red spikenard, vetiver, white lotus
Second (svadhishthana/sacral)	Agarwood, blood orange, blue chamomile, cardamom, galangal, jasmine, massoia bark, neroli, patchouli, pink pepper seed, red spikenard, vanilla, white lotus
Third (manipura/solar plexus)	Betel leaf, black pepper, blood orange, cardamom, elemi, kaffir lime leaf, lemon, pine, pink pepper seed, red spikenard, vetiver, white lotus
Fourth (anahata/heart)	Kaffir lime leaf, massoia bark, neroli, pine, red spikenard, rose, rosewood, white lotus
Fifth (vishuddha/throat)	Agarwood, betel leaf, blue chamomile, elemi, frankincense, lavender, red spikenard, white lotus
Sixth (ajna/third eye)	Jasmine, lemon, red spikenard, sandalwood, white lotus
Seventh (sahaswara/crown)	Chinese rice flower, lime, red spikenard, rose, white lotus

Essential Oils for Purification

Although all essential oils create positive shifts, the three listed below are especially dynamic for deep purification. Use any time your energetic, emotional, or mental body feels gummed up. These oils also have a long tradition of purifying the physical body. As part of a spiritual practice, many people use these essential oils in a monthly ceremony for a general reset. They are also recommended as the first step in any intense healing journey.

HEMLOCK SPRUCE
(*Tsuga canadensis*)

Element: Ether, with seed of earth

Key Traits: A grounded, elevated nature; cooperation; peace; purification; protection; joy; tranquillity; humility; self-reliance; fortitude;

and a profound sense of the spiritual. An emanation of the divine masculine.

Divine Archetype: Great Spirit/Grandfather (peace, wisdom, tranquillity)

Hemlock spruce essential oil is used for achieving a grounded, elevated state and for establishing shelter from discordant energy. It also imparts the energy of fortitude and firm self-reliance. In his book *The Meaning of Trees,* Fred Hageneder beautifully describes some of the energy surrounding this magnificent tree.

> The spruce is also the centre of sacred teachings among the indigenous tribes of southern Canada, who call it the Peace Tree. Its lessons are: to co-operate and exchange with other life forms; to be connected to the earth and the heavens; and to exhibit a joyful and tranquil humility.[4]

Shamans of the Tsimshian tribe in the Pacific Northwest also used spruce boughs during purification rituals. According to Hageneder, most Native American tribes believed that spruce offers protection from damaging influences.

TULSI
(Ocimum sanctum)

Element: Fire, with seed of air

Key Traits: Blueprint of the perfected self, understanding what the act of devotion means, pure unobstructed/unconditional love, purification and protection. An emanation of divine masculine.

Divine Archetype: Krishna (the eighth incarnation of Vishnu)

A sacred plant of India and beloved of Krishna (the embodiment of love and of the divine joy that destroys all pain), tulsi, sometimes called holy basil, is *sattvic* in nature (meaning that it embodies the perfected principle of light, perception, and harmony). Use this essential oil to purify and protect the energy of yourself and/or your environment. Tulsi opens and heals the heart chakra, teaching the true energy of loving detachment and devotion.

Caution: Not for use with pregnancy.

WHITE BIRCH
(*Betula alba*)

Element: Water, with seed of fire

Key Traits: Bringing light into the darkness, deep purification, expanding your appreciation of beauty and your own inner radiance, emotional succor, protection and a profound sense of calm. An expression of the divine feminine.

Divine Archetypes: Brigid; Lady of the Forest/White Goddess

Birch has been traditionally used in Native American sweat-lodge ceremonies, whose purpose is deep purification of the spirit (subtle bodies). The essential oil can be used with the same intent to cleanse and purify. The essential oil of birch has the same effect on the spirit as the living tree has in dreary winter landscapes, bringing radiance into the darkness. This essential oil also enhances your ability to experience beauty and remain calm.

Fred Hageneder tells us:

Named after the whiteness of its bark, the birch tree shares its name with the ancient Irish goddess Brigid, both names deriving from the Indo-European word bder(e)g, "shining white."[5]

In Russian folklore, as well as in Norse and Germanic cultures, the birch itself is called Lady of the Forest. Many cultures attribute qualities of nurturing, mothering, renewal, and protection to the white birch tree. The nourishing, caring birch is an age-old symbol of the White Goddess, and the Germanic rune *berkana*, "birch," stands in part for protection.

7
Choosing and Using Essential Oils

One of the most delightful aspects of working with essential oils is deciding how you will choose the oils that are right for your situation, how you will use them, and the proper preparation of the oils. There are so many options, and all are valuable.

Choosing Essential Oils

You could approach the question of how to choose which essential oil to work with by many avenues. Following are a few examples.

+ **Problem solving.** In this case, you are aware of the issue you want to solve or the state of being you want to cultivate, so you simply choose the oil(s) that support this goal and build a practice around them.
+ **Archetypal energy.** You identify which archetypal energy you want to work with and make an essential oil blend and ritual to invoke that energy.
+ **Oracle and antidote method.** The phrase "oracle and antidote" means that the vibrations of the essential oils can tell you which oil you need (oracle) to improve your situation (antidote). What you're feeling for here is resonance: the essential oil you need will

resonate with the disharmonious energy you would like to untangle. This method is itself a form of healing ritual, and we'll talk more about it in chapter 11.

There are, of course, other methods of choosing essential oils, and you should use the method that feels right to you. There are also many methods of employing essential oils in healing rituals. We'll get into the specifics in part 3, but for now let's talk about the very basics of using essential oils.

Methods for Using Essential Oils

When employing essential oils for ritual use, the following are the most common vehicles.

+ **Personal anointing:** Applying the essential oil to the body in a targeted area
+ **Ritual object anointing:** Applying the essential oil to an object, like an amulet, to amplify its energy or to sanctify it
+ **Massage:** Massaging an essential oil (blended with a base oil) on oneself or another in a targeted area or over the entire body
+ **Ritual bathing:** Using an essential oil in a fragrant/vibrational-healing bath
+ **Diffusion:** Using a diffuser to disperse an essential oil into the air
+ **Misters:** Using a fine mist atomizer to blend essential oils and water for use as a spray for the aura, for anointing objects, or for elsewhere in your environment

Dosages and Dilutions

Everything is poisonous, and nothing is without poison.
The dose alone prevents something from being a poison.

PARACELSUS

The following dilution ratios are standard in the aromatherapy field. I suggest starting with half the recommended dosage and observing how your body responds, then adjusting the ratio of essential oil to base oil from there.

Note: Always use massoia bark in half dosages or lower, and perform a skin patch test before topical use. If skin irritation occurs even at a low dosage, discontinue use topically and enjoy massoia only for diffusion and the ritual anointing of objects.

FULL-BODY APPLICATION

Dilution: 3 to 5 drops of essential oil in 1 teaspoon of base oil; 7 to 25 drops in 1 ounce of base oil; or 20 to 60 drops in 3½ ounces of base oil.

These ratios are guidelines for *massage blends* or *full-body application*. Each individual is different; some people require an even lower blend ratio, while others benefit from a more concentrated dose.

LOCALIZED RITUAL ANOINTING OF THE BODY

Dilution: 4 to 7 drops of essential oil in 1 teaspoon of base oil; or 7 to 18 drops in 1 tablespoon of base oil.

These are more concentrated blends that will be applied only to specific body areas, with a focus on scent. Every individual is different, so always be mindful of dosage and how your body responds, and adjust the ratio of essential oil to base oil accordingly.

RITUAL ANOINTING OF AN OBJECT

Dilution: 1 drop of essential oil in 1 to 3 tablespoons of base oil, depending on the reactivity of the surface you are anointing.

Always test a small, unseen area first. Once you have determined the appropriate ratio, anoint the object you are working with as you ruminate on the energy you are invoking. If you are anointing jewelry, when you are finished, gently buff your piece to a shine with a clean, soft cloth.

RITUAL BATHS

Dilution: 1 to 13 drops of essential oil* (always be mindful of how it affects you, and adjust the ratios as needed) in one of the following bases.

+ 3 tablespoons of a base oil (see chapter 8)
+ 1 cup of milk (animal, coconut, soy, rice, etc.; milk's general energy is nourishing, nurturing, loving, cushioning, and fostering)
+ ½ to 1 cup of sea salt or Epsom salts with 1 tablespoon of base oil added (salt's general energy is purifying, cleansing, clearing, and detoxifying)
+ ½ cup of milk and ½ cup of salt blended together (this combination supports the clearing away of disharmonic patterns that may hamper the new energetic seedlings you are nurturing to fruition)

Essential oils are highly volatile and not water soluble, so a base is needed to stabilize them before you add them to a foot, hand, or full-immersion bath. Combine the essential oils with your chosen base, run a bath, then add the essential oil blend and stir to mix it into the water.

DIFFUSION

For any aromatherapy diffuser, follow the manufacturer's instructions for dilution and use. Depending on which tattva you intend to invoke, you may want to use a specific type of diffuser.

+ Earth: Any style of diffuser, as scent stimulates the earth element
+ Water: Water-based mister
+ Fire: Tea light diffuser
+ Air: Aromatherapy nebulizer
+ Ether: Aromatherapy nebulizer

---

*Note that this method of application is not recommended for massoia bark.

MISTERS

One of the joys of creating misters is the creative freedom it allows. You may choose to blend for fragrance or for numerological meaning. You can literally use as much or as little oil as you would like, because this application only affects your olfactory system and energetic body and these offer no contraindications. So play with dilution ratios until you find what feels delicious to you.

Use a glass bottle (that is not clear) with a fine atomizer. In a 1-ounce bottle, for example, add 1 tablespoon of witch hazel or alcohol and the essential oil(s) you wish to use. A good rule of thumb for a starting point is 45 drops of oil. Top with the purest water you have access to, recap your bottle, and gently shake it. This is a good time to set intentions, use a mantra, or apply a label with a yantra you created.

Using Essential Oils Wisely

✦ If you do not know how your body will respond to a certain essential oil, dosage, and dilution rate, perform a skin patch test first: Prepare the dilution you would like to work with, apply this solution to the inside crook of your elbow, and wait for twenty-four hours. If no irritation occurs, you may use the essential oil in the dosage you applied.

✦ For those essential oils that you know carry a risk of causing a bad reaction, like massoia bark, perform a patch test, use them at a high dilution rate and a low dosage, and be aware of the symptoms of a negative reaction.

✦ Always dilute essential oils properly before use. Very few essential oils are intended to be used "neat," or without being diluted. In fact, there are no benefits to applying oils neat, and neat usage can even compromise the beneficial healing properties of the essential oil being used. Essential oils are highly concentrated materials. If used neat it can result in contact dermatitis and sensitization (this lasts for life, meaning you can never use the oil that caused the reaction again or any oils that share a similar chemical makeup). Additionally, the fatty base oils you blend your essential oils in offer a wide range of benefits physically and energetically.

+ If an essential oil causes your skin to feel itchy or irritated, quell the feeling by applying a fatty base oil, natural lotion, aloe gel, full-fat milk, or mashed cucumber pulp to the affected area. Follow up with an oatmeal bath. Discontinue topical use of the offending essential oil for five to thirty days, depending on the severity of the reaction. In extreme cases, from that point forward reserve that essential oil for ritual anointing of objects or diffusion.

+ If any other sensitivity to an essential oil occurs, such as difficulty breathing, dizziness, or another condition of concern, see your health care provider at once.

+ Essential oils should not come into contact with your eyes and ears, and do not take them internally. Do not administer them to children, the elderly, or the frail, even topically and diluted, unless under the supervision of your health care provider. Use with a mister or diffuser is safe for all.

+ Track your energetic progress by taking off one week per month from your practice, ceasing the use of any type of physical or ritual application. This allows your body and energy field to recalibrate and reset, thereby giving you an unambiguous reading of your current energetic state when it does not have outside support. When you pick up your practice again, you can clearly understand what is needed to fine-tune your practice to support your highest growth.

Always be mindful of how your body reacts. These are only guidelines.

8

Choosing and Using Base Oils

Like essential oils, base oils have their own unique vibrational patterns and healing qualities. Base oils and essential oils can be paired energetically so that the energetic pattern of the base oil supports that of the essential oil. Take as an example a case in which you wish to address patterns of being bound by ego or displeasure with your personal physical appearance and the difficulties associated with these thought patterns. These emotional conditions are in part associated with the fire element, which, when out of balance, usually manifests as maladies that are intensely self-focused. In the physical body an out-of-balance fire energy gives rise to physical conditions such as skin irritations, inflammation, and oily skin. Thus, you would look for a base oil that helps bring these "hot," fire-based conditions into balance in combination with an essential oil that supports the desired shift in your energetic pattern.

The essential oil of betel leaf helps heal ego-based imbalances and shift habituated ways of being. Almond oil, on the physical level, is a light oil that helps soothe inflammation and irritated skin, making it a good base for massage blends. On a deeper level, almond oil addresses ego-based issues that specifically deal with aging, beauty, and how you identify with your physical appearance. Almond helps heal the fear of growing old, helps you accept with grace the aging process, and aids you in perceiving beauty beyond simple physical appearance. Thus, a blend of betel leaf essential oil with almond base oil will dynamically assist in addressing unbalanced elemental fire issues that manifest as ego distortions.

The more aware you become of personal disharmonic patterns and the tools offered as antidotes, the more successfully and dynamically you can shift these patterns. In this hypothetical case, the ego-grasping issue is an attachment to physical appearance and the resulting fear of aging. Almond cannot be used as an essential oil, as it is toxic when distilled, so a healthy alternative is to use it as the base oil for the blend, creating a synergy between the betel leaf and almond. The result is a more precisely tuned energetic pattern.

Base Oils: Profiles

ALMOND OIL, SWEET
(*Prunus dulcis*)

Energetic Signature: *Vitality.* Helps arrest the fear of aging and makes the passage of time sacred and not solely experienced through the physical body. Opens you to the complex beauty of self and a strong inner vitality.

Practical Use: A nourishing demulcent (relieving irritation; soothing) that is most similar to the skin's own natural oil (sebum). Its light aroma makes it an ideal base for massage blends. Can be used to address eczema.

APRICOT KERNEL OIL
(*Prunus armeniaca*)

Energetic Signature: *Balance.* Helps balance mood swings and extreme emotional states. Promotes exchange between the mental and subtle bodies. Facilitates the reconciliation of internal conflicts and strong negative emotions that have been stored in the body. It empowers you to take responsibility in your life and make the changes necessary for health and well-being. Also helps foster delight in life itself.

Practical Use: A nourishing medium-weight oil that is good for dry skin and leaves no residue. It makes a nice massage or anointing base, as it has almost no scent. High in vitamins A and C.

AVOCADO OIL
(Persea gratissima)

Energetic Signature: *Positive touch.* Harmonizes the body and mind by dissolving emotional tension and the negative influence of past pain that causes you to turn inward and harden against love that is being offered. Offers shelter when you are feeling overwhelmed with emotion. Avocado allows you to become more vulnerable to others without fear and facilitates intimacy and healing through touch.

Practical Use: A thick, luxurious, heavy oil with a strong, earthy, green scent. This oil is highly penetrating and deeply moisturizing. High in oleic acid, linoleic acid, lecithin, and vitamin D. It can be beneficial for hard-to-heal sores, eczema, and dry or mature skin.

COCONUT OIL
(Cocos nucifera)

Energetic Signature: *Endurance.* Promotes endurance and perseverance for completing tasks, which in turn helps you manifest your full potential. Also helps provide strong, steady energy and the ability to welcome challenges and be solution oriented.

Practical Use: A thick oil that is semisolid at room temperature but melts easily on the body and feels good while doing so! It is greasy when applied but forms a readily absorbable anointing base.

CORN OIL
(*Zea mays*)

Energetic Signature: *Fertility.* Supports alignment with earth energies, opening you to the *corn*ucopia that life offers. Helps usher in abundance on all levels, especially the joy and pleasure associated with the feminine. Supports increased creativity and birthing the projects that follow. Useful for fostering friendships based on mutual support and growth and promoting synergy to achieve goals larger than yourself.

Practical Use: A moderately viscous oil with a faint scent.

PART 3

Healing Practices

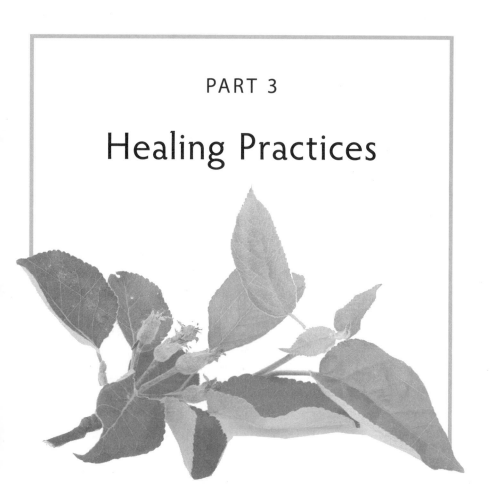

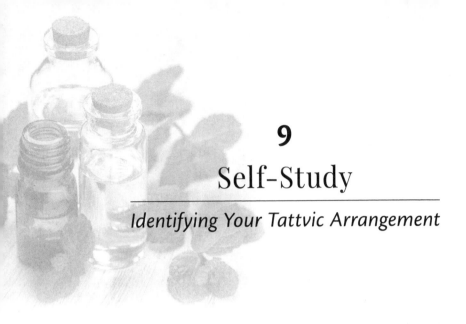

9
Self-Study

Identifying Your Tattvic Arrangement

Our personal interaction with the world is a radically subjective experience. Some people like the color yellow best, while others prefer a different color; some people like the taste of cilantro, while others detest it; some people experience a "fight" response to stress, while others experience a "flight" response. We each perceive, categorize, and react to our environment in different ways, guided largely by the following three factors.

+ Birth karma, or the specific arrangement of tattvic influences on our mental and emotional patterns
+ Samskaras, or the inherited energetic imprints or thoughtforms that guide our mental and emotional patterns
+ Cultural influences, or the collective social paradigms that shape our mental and emotional patterns

Recognizing and understanding each tattva's signature—the ways in which it influences our subconscious mental and emotional conditioning—opens the door to working with all aspects of the self, including birth karma, samskaras, and cultural influences. As the word *subconscious* suggests, there are aspects of the self that operate below our level of awareness. Intentional self-study, while valuable, only allows us to view what we are already conscious of; we need a means of examining the patterns that are hidden from plain view. Like a record groove singing out what has been scored into it, our mental and emotional patterns reveal the influence of the tattvas in our energetic continuum.

The Rise and Fall of Tattvic Influences

The Caterpillar and Alice looked at each other for some time in silence; at last the Caterpillar took the hookah out of its mouth, and addressed her in a languid, sleepy voice.

"Who are you?" said the Caterpillar.

This was not an encouraging opening for a conversation. Alice replied, rather shyly, "I—I hardly know, sir, just at present—at least I know who I was when I got up this morning, but I think I must have been changed several times since then."

"What do you mean by that?" said the Caterpillar sternly. "Explain yourself!"

"I can't explain myself, *I'm afraid, sir," said Alice, "because I'm not myself, you see."*

"I don't see," said the Caterpillar.

"I'm afraid I can't put it more clearly," Alice replied very politely, "for I can't understand it myself to begin with; and being so many different sizes in a day is very confusing."

"It isn't," said the Caterpillar.

"Well, perhaps you haven't found it so yet," said Alice; "but when you have to turn into a chrysalis—you will some day, you know—and then after that into a butterfly, I should think you'll feel it a little queer, won't you?"

"Not a bit," said the Caterpillar.

"Well, perhaps your *feelings may be different,"* said
Alice; *"all I know is, it would feel very queer to* me."
   "You!" said *the Caterpillar contemptuously. "Who are*
you?"

Alice's Adventures in Wonderland,
by Lewis Carroll

"Who are you?" That is a good question indeed, and Alice's answer
holds a significant revelation: we are not static creatures. We are always
flowing among the different elements as their influence on us rises and
falls, waxes and wanes, builds and retreats. Some tattvic influences
shape long-term conditioning and ingrained patterns of behavior, while
others present as short-term or fleeting impulses.

Whatever their longevity, our sensory experience is determined by
how the elements manifest within us at any particular time. The elements are the filter through which we experience life; they shape our
perception of the world. The caterpillar's combination of constituent
elements supports metamorphosis, or growth and radical change from
one stage to the next, making the idea of undergoing such transformation easy and natural (earth transformed by fire into air). For Alice,
the experience of such radical change is very unsettling (earth wanting
to remain earth). This is a classic earth response: the desire to remain
"entrenched" in a way of being.*

The ability to gracefully participate in the flow of life and to be
present in the moment at hand is paramount to authentic growth. A
wise individual does not attempt to live in the boneyard of yesterday's
experiences. Many Native American tribes speak of "dragging your old
bones around," referring to the pattern of holding on to old stories and
outmoded ways of being because they feel familiar, because we feel obli-
gated to uphold tradition, or for any reason that keeps us chained to a
specific way of being that no longer serves our highest growth.

---

*Alice's physical traits (having blond, thick, straight hair; large blue eyes; and a round
figure) indicate that she is a classic kapha (earth/water).

The idea of "self" as malleable and ever-changing can be disorienting for some, but once we understand it, we can objectively observe the element(s) present in our self at a given point and interpret the effects on a personal level. Without understanding our own unique elemental combination, it is difficult to understand the deep causation patterns that dominate the subconscious self and to choose the appropriate vibrational tools for healing.

Just like humans, plants have physical markers that identify their elemental composition. This concept, known as the "doctrine of signatures," means that the exterior of the plant expresses what the interior holds. For example, yellow and orange fruits and vegetables generally contain beta-carotene, zeaxanthin, flavonoids, lycopene, potassium, and vitamin C. White fruits and vegetables generally contain nutrients such as beta-glucans, epigallocatechin gallate, and lignans with powerful immune-boosting activity. Early alchemists taught that star-shaped flowers generally have a cosmic orientation and offer support with spiritual lessons, whereas bell-shaped flowers that point downward generally address issues of embodiment, grounding, and soul life. This system of identification is analogous to recognizing that a redhead (a fire type) will probably have a strong left-brain orientation, or that a person with large, sensuous eyes (a water type) will probably have a strong emotional IQ.

All of the healing tools we find in nature—plants, minerals, metals, and stones—have their own unique arrangement of constituents, from basic chemical properties to tattvic influences. Energetically, they work like vibrational keys to the energetic mechanisms inside us and can help us unlock our potential. As with any key and lock, one must employ the correct key to gain the desired access. I have had clients who insisted that flower essences or essential oils did not work for them. It took a bit of explaining to convince them that a vibrational remedy must be precisely tuned to the disharmonic energy being addressed for any effect to occur. For example, the healing signatures of devil's claw and red rose both address sexual energy, but they work on different patterns. The vibrational essence of devil's claw balances the disharmonic pattern of using personal magnetism or attractiveness to manipulate others, whereas the vibrational essence of red rose cultivates boldness and passion. People frequently get caught up in using "rescue remedies" or popular essential oils like tea tree as a cure-all. These remedies are perfect for their intended purpose, but they most definitely do not cover all energetic maladies. It is vital to understand your personal elemental signature, the root energy that needs to be addressed, and the energy pattern of the essential oils or vibrational essences you are using to experience dynamic, directed results.

Identifying Active Tattvas and Chakras

Knowing which elements and chakras are active in our lives is most beneficial to self-study. As Harish Johari—a brilliant yogi who specialized in the tantric arts—notes, "One should become *tattvadarshi* (an observer of the elements) because all physiological and psychological changes arise from the mutation of . . . the *tattvas,* or elements."[1]

To identify which tattva is dominant and active at any given time, you can use the Yoni Mudra. Johari provides the following description.

Place the right and left thumbs on the openings of the ears and press them shut; with the middle fingers of each hand, one should close the two nostrils. Then place the two index fingers on closed eyelids and apply a little pressure. With the two remaining fingers—the third finger and the little finger of both hands—one should tightly close the lips.

Before doing Yoni Mudra, one should take a full, deep breath. After a while, colors will begin to emerge. The process is facilitated by increasing the pressure on the eyelids.

- The presence of yellow denotes the Earth element.
- The presence of white indicates the Water element.
- The presence of red indicates the Fire element.

- The presence of smoky green or black indicates the Air element.
- When one sees small dots of many colors, the presence of Akasha [ether] is indicated.[2]

You can also simply close your eyes, cup them with your palms to block out all light, and wait to see what color of internal light arises. Often you will find that more than one color is present.

Like the tattvas, the chakras have colors that indicate which center is active and presenting itself.

+ The presence of glowing red denotes the root (first) chakra.
+ The presence of bright orange denotes the sensual/inner child (second) chakra.
+ The presence of radiant yellow indicates the inner sun (third) chakra.
+ The presence of vibrant, electric green or pink indicates the heart (fourth) chakra.
+ The presence of vivid blue indicates the throat (fifth) chakra.
+ The presence of rich indigo indicates the third eye (sixth) chakra.
+ The presence of radiant white or violet indicates the crown (seventh) chakra.

My personal experience has been that chakra colors tend to be more vivid and tattva colors more matte. Yellow, for example, could signify either the inner sun (third) chakra or the earth element. If the yellow is luminous and shines like the sun, it is probably the third chakra; if the yellow is duller with a golden hue, it is most likely the earth element. Similarly, the element air presents itself as a matte smoky green, while the fourth chakra presents a vibrant, almost electric green.

Personal karmic influences create slight variations in how each of us perceives the tattvas and chakras. I myself see both green and pink for the heart chakra, and I have learned that, for me, green represents a transcendent love, while pink denotes a love that needs anchoring in a specific action. The task is to become familiar with the symbolic language of the elements and how *you* distinguish each one.

The more you work with the tattvas, the easier it becomes to tune in to their energetic influence on you. Eventually you will no longer need to do the Yoni Mudra to see which element is active; you will simply close your eyes and observe in a snap which colors are active. Eventually, as you nurture your connection with the tattvas, the primordial tattva shapes (see chapter 3) will start to present themselves along with the colors.

Learning the Language of Tattvas

Ritual bathing with essential oils is one way to familiarize yourself with the symbolic language of the tattvas—the colors, shapes, and vibrations they present to you. Draw a warm bath in a darkened room. After you are in the bath, add a few drops of an essential oil to the bathwater or mist the room with a diluted essential oil spray. If the room is pitch dark, you can keep your eyes open; otherwise close them. You might receive a "flash" of color as you energetically come into contact with the energy of the oil. This is a wonderful way to find out how individual elements present themselves to you. Lying still and submerged in a darkened room helps you tune in to the amplified vibration of an essential oil and the elements to which it is linked.

Balancing the Tattvas

It is tempting to think of tattvas, chakras, and doshas solely in abstract terms. In truth, however, they are the silent motivators for all you do. The more you explore your personal makeup, the less likely you are to be manipulated by your elemental components. For example, I am a vata/kapha type, and within that I evolve more from air, ether, and water and lack much earth. I do not have much fire in my makeup. The way I process is heavily influenced by this elemental arrangement. I am naturally very creative and intuitive (air/ether/water), have a healthy inner child (water/air), and am drawn to work with the emotions (water/air) and the subtle self (ether). I also dread routine (air) and have a hard time getting my ideas out of my mind and onto paper (air) but easily translate concepts into daily practice (water).

Because that elemental combination is not always beneficial, I employ many tools to help me energetically craft my elemental makeup so that I can live a life of balance. The foundational concept we are exploring is to create a balance within the self. Because I do not naturally have much fire or earth in my makeup, I must stimulate these energies when needed and feed balancing energy into my water, air, and ether aspects; otherwise I will flitter about endlessly without finishing projects, as I become bored and then float to my next idea.

I can bring my body into balance with vibrational tools and rituals that cultivate fire and earth energy. Fire energy gives rise to dynamic action and sharp intellect (ruling the left brain and conventional intelligence); earth energy gives rise to stability and endurance. Together these energies counterbalance the dominating effect of water, air, and ether on my natural elemental constitution.

As a more specific example, the shadow side of my air makeup includes being shy to the point of hiding. It is one of my most significant elemental challenges. Fire energy brings with it the bravery required for exposing the self. When I work to cultivate fire energy, this vibration helps me overcome the bondage of personally imposed limitations—thoughts like "I could never do that," "That is out of my league," or "What if they don't like my idea?" Fire energy severs those negative energetic cords.

Once you have become familiar with your own tattvic arrangement and the subtle tides of influence that the tattvas have upon your mental and emotional patterns, you can begin to work directly with them for balance, healing, and positive growth. Chapter 10 discusses the tools, delivery methods, and rituals that invoke each tattva on your journey toward energetic balance and spiritual growth.

Elemental Quiz

Circle the numbered item that most appeals to you from each category.

I delight in

1. Walking barefoot on the earth
2. Swimming or taking baths
3. Competitive sports or puzzles
4. Loving touch (i.e., holding hands, snuggling, bodywork)
5. Conversations

My favorite sense to explore the world with is

1. Fragrance
2. Taste
3. Sight
4. Touch
5. Sound

I would like to manifest in my life

1. Creating abundance
2. Developing my creativity
3. Sharpening my intellect
4. Experiencing true love
5. Having a profound knowing of life's purpose

The color I am most drawn to is

1. Red
2. Orange
3. Yellow
4. Green or pink
5. Black or blue

What verse moves you most?

1. *Expect your every need to be met. Expect the answer to every problem, expect abundance on every level.* —Eileen Caddy

2. *Your sexuality is god's love letter to you, a miracle of biological engineering that could have been devised only by a mind of vast and humorous generosity, a mind that knew the pain and the sense of confinement earthly beings would feel and wanted to make sure you might always have glimpses of heaven.*
   —Jalaja Bonheim

3. *Knowing others is intelligence; knowing yourself is true wisdom. Mastering others is strength; mastering yourself is true power.*
   —Lao-tzu

4. *Love has no desire but to fulfill itself. To melt and be like a running brook that sings its melody to the night. To wake at dawn with a winged heart and give thanks for another day of loving.* —Kahlil Gibran

5. *Keep your thoughts positive because your thoughts become your words. Keep your words positive because your words become your behaviors. Keep your behaviors positive because your behaviors become your habits. Keep your habits positive because your habits become your values. Keep your values positive because your values become your destiny.* —Gandhi

I most struggle with

1. Feeling a sense of lack
2. Living a soulful life
3. Maintaining a positive sense of self
4. Being able to forgive
5. Sitting for meditation

I most fear

1. Being responsible for my day-to-day life
2. My sexuality
3. Confrontation
4. Opening my heart to another
5. Speaking my truth

I desire to heal

1. My use of sex, drugs, food, or other substances so as to feel
2. My wounded emotions or my need to keep my thoughts and feelings hidden from others
3. My inability to express my own desires or my need to use force to control others
4. My feelings of vulnerability and rejection or my inability to allow others in
5. My failure to fully actualize my spiritual gifts

I most want to cultivate

1. Body knowledge, instinctual knowing, and stability of self
2. Sensuality, sexual intimacy, and giving and receiving pleasure
3. Action, authority, integrity, personal power, and radiance
4. Union with others and self and the transformation of the common into the divine
5. Spiritual gifts such as clairvoyance, clairaudience, being a clear channel, et cetera

I want to invite into my life

1. A pragmatic, practical nature that allows me to get things done
2. Work with dreams, deep mystery, archetypes, and cycles for growth
3. A capacity to initiate projects, passion, enthusiasm, and growth
4. Positive change, active dreaming, and visualization of what could be
5. The ability to be a brilliant orator, using my words to shape my reality

The relationship I crave most is

1. A fertile home life: children, partner, garden, pets, et cetera
2. A passionate love affair that stimulates my deepest creativity
3. A partner who stimulates my highest potential
4. Love that is sweet and nurturing yet offers freedom
5. One with a spiritual teacher

Add up the number of items you circled from each row.

1. Earth: _3_____
2. Water: _5_____
3. Fire: _2_____
4. Air: _4_____
5. Ether: _5_____

The results of the quiz show you which elemental aspects in your life your deep self could like to cultivate. Pay attention to the top one or two elements, and focus working with these elements to help you develop the area of life associated with those vibrations.

Water & Ether

10

Deepening Connections

Working with the Tattvas

As we have established, the tattvas are active principles that are "alive" not just in our subconscious but in our entire physical and energetic continuum. Simply gazing upon a tattva's archetypal image (the shape and color that carry its vibrational signature), speaking its sacred sound, or absorbing its frequency from an associated essential oil or other vibrational tool stimulates all of the qualities associated with that tattva. A golden yellow square, for example, is a numinous shape and color combination that resonates with the energy of the earth tattva at our deepest levels.

Stimulation can refer either to amplification of positive aspects or purification by removing negative traits. *Purification* is the ceremonial or spiritual act of cleansing. Thus, in working with the tattvas, stimulation and purification are two different ways of looking at the same process.

Swami Satyasangananda has an interesting comment concerning this process.

The causal level constituted by the tattwas is the most difficult to purify because it does not come under the influence of the conscious mind and thought. It requires a powerful force of concentrated energy to create a transformation on this level. This is attainable in tattwa shuddhi through repetition of the tattwa bija mantras [sacred sounds] and visualization of their respective yantras [sacred geometry]. These have a profound influence on the causal body and unconscious mind, and are able to purge the deep-rooted samskaras [inherited thoughtforms] and archetypes that obscure the experience of unlimited consciousness.[1]

Meditation is a powerful tool for achieving transformation at this causal level, because it allows you to work with energy beyond the reach of the mind and thoughts, focusing on the yantra (sacred symbol), mantra (sacred sound), and essential oils that resonate with the tattva being invoked. It attunes you to the vibration needed to address the causal body. Regarding the causal body, Vedic master David Frawley tells us that

the causal body functions during deep sleep and profound meditation, during which we live in our own consciousness devoid of external objects, perceived or imaginary. The causal body is not located as a form or an impression in space and time, but exists as idea that creates time and space according to its qualities.[2]

To balance the tattvas, it is generally deemed most beneficial to work from the grossest to the subtlest element—that is, from earth to ether. You might also simply work with whichever element presents itself to you for your attention. Work in a cycle, invoking first earth, then water, fire, air, and finally ether, in the visualizations described below. After completing the cycle several times, when the elements feel awakened, ask which element you need to focus on. Once an element reveals itself, choose the corresponding tools, delivery methods, and rituals to support your work with that element.

If you are feeling unbalanced or stuck, check to see which element is active (see chapter 9). Look to see what behaviors may be running amok when that element is out of balance—that is, the "shadow" properties of the tattvas (see chapter 3). Then utilize the proper tools and rituals to help bring balance.

All of the rituals and activities discussed in this book bring balance to your energetic patterns. There are many healing systems out there that focus on diverting energy, but my system of vibrational healing is entirely about balance. If a particular energy is too dense, the practices in this book will lighten it. If it is anemic, they will fortify it. Your job is to become familiar with your own unique energetic pattern, to identify inharmonious energies, and to work with the tools and rituals herein—essential oils, mantras, yantras, and so on—to assist in dissolving calcified causation patterns and laying down new behavioral patterns that support your highest self.

Working with Earth

This is the foundational stage in which we stabilize the body, which is the fulcrum of consciousness. This stage includes all activities that support physical health, including ritual bathing, scented massage, and ritual anointing. It also includes exercise, yoga, breathing exercises, a healthy diet, and any other practice that supports balance in the physical body.

VIBRATIONAL TOOLS

Aromas can improve performance and capacity to remember, they can make you alert, or relaxed, and change your mood.

VALERIE ANN WORWOOD,
THE FRAGRANT MIND

+ **Sense:** Earth is primarily stimulated by smell. Seek out scents that stimulate the states of being you seek and support your mood, state of mind, and energy.
+ **Essential oils:** Use essential oils that emanate from earth (first chakra), galangal, or massoia bark. Any style of diffuser is suitable for stimulating earth; the form of diffusion matters less than the scent of the essential oil you use.
+ **Metal:** Wear copper.

MEDITATION

To begin, invoke the earth element; see the box below. Next, settle into a comfortable seated or reclined position and close your eyes. Visualize a golden yellow square extending from your feet to your knees, all the while repeating *lam* silently in your mind. Inhale any earth-based fragrance you have used, and feel the vibration from any anointing oil. Look for the matte yellow behind your eyelids, indicating that the earth element is present. Breathe slowly and deeply. Maintain the visualization for anywhere from one to twenty minutes. This seemingly simple act stimulates the purification process of the earth tattva.

Invoking a Tattva

Any meditation to stimulate the purification of a tattva should begin with an invocation of that tattva to set your intention. You might speak its sacred syllable aloud, or you might anoint the associated chakra with an essential oil that stimulates that tattva (see chapter 3 for details on which chakras are linked to which tattvas). Alternatively, you might use that tattva-stimulating essential oil to make a mister (see chapter 7) and use it to mist your aura, or you could use that essential oil in a bath, an aromatherapy diffuser, or a tea light diffuser, depending on which element you are working with.

Working with Water

Water rules the emotions, dreams, and soul. Keeping a dream journal, engaging in emotionally edifying conversations, and seeking out creative expression are wonderful ways to work with this energy.

Your food choices can greatly affect elemental water energy in your body. You may want to work with a dietitian, macrobiotic practitioner, or ayurvedic guide if you need clarification on what foods are best for your body type (dosha).

VIBRATIONAL TOOLS

People who love to eat are always the best people.

JULIA CHILD

+ **Sense:** Water is primarily stimulated by taste. Consume organic, healthful, seasonal food appropriate for your body type and, on occasion, food that is so tasty it melts your soul.
+ **Essential oils:** Use essential oils that emanate from water (second chakra), agarwood, galangal, or massoia bark. A water-based mister and aromatherapeutic baths are especially dynamic for invoking this element.
+ **Metal:** Wear silver.

MEDITATION

To begin, invoke the water element; see the box on the previous page. Then take a comfortable seated or reclined position and close your eyes. Visualize a recumbent white or silver crescent moon materializing in the space between your knees and your navel, all the while silently repeating water's mantra, *vam*. Work with this image for one to twenty minutes.

Working with Fire

Fire rules conventional intelligence, competition, and mastering a skill. This energy thrives when you are participating in competitive or goal-oriented events, from working crossword puzzles to rebuilding an engine to learning a classical art like piano or fencing.

VIBRATIONAL TOOLS

Look at the trees, look at the birds, look at the clouds, look at the stars . . . and if you have eyes you will be able to see that the whole existence is joyful.

OSHO

+ **Sense:** Fire is primarily stimulated by sight. Practice sacred geometry meditation (page 140), use color to stimulate a specific response, gaze upon sacred images such as thangkas or mandalas, and look upon pristine nature or inspirational structures.
+ **Essential oils:** Use essential oils that emanate from fire (third chakra), betel leaf, or kaffir lime leaf. A tea light diffuser is especially dynamic for invoking this element.
+ **Metal:** Wear gold.

MEDITATION

To begin, invoke the fire element; see the box on page 135. Then settle into a comfortable seated or reclined position and close your eyes. Visualize a red triangle in the area from your navel to your heart, all the while silently repeating fire's mantra, *ram*. Work with this energy for one to twenty minutes.

Working with Air

Air promotes curiosity, freedom from attachments, and shifting consciousness. Try lying on your back and gazing in to the sky as you feel the wind on your skin, allowing your mind to wander, and enjoy daydreaming.

VIBRATIONAL TOOLS

The way to health is to have a . . . scented massage every day.

HIPPOCRATES

+ **Sense:** Air is primarily stimulated by touch. Enjoy massage therapy (self-massage or from a therapist) and ritual anointing with essential oils. Use your skin to absorb nature's pharmacy.

+ **Essential oils:** Use essential oils that emanate from air (fourth chakra), kaffir lime leaf, or massoia bark. An aromatherapy nebulizer is especially dynamic for invoking this element.
+ **Metal:** Wear silver.

MEDITATION

To begin, invoke the air element; see the box on page 135. Then settle into a comfortable seated or reclined position and close your eyes. Visualize a large green-gray circle formed in the area of your heart. Silently repeat air's mantra, *yam*. Work with this visualization for one to twenty minutes.

Working with Ether

Ether is the gateway to the divine and is used primarily for spiritual pursuits.

VIBRATIONAL TOOLS

Music is the mediator between the life of the senses and the life of the spirit.

BEETHOVEN

+ **Sense:** Ether is primarily stimulated by sound. Sing, listen to, or chant mantras; read scriptures or affirmations aloud; listen to sounds from nature or any inspiring music; or enjoy a healing session from a professional sound healer.

+ **Essential oils:** Use essential oils that emanate from ether (fifth chakra), agarwood, or betel leaf. An aromatherapy nebulizer is especially dynamic for invoking this element.

+ **Metal:** Wear anointed silver jewelry.

MEDITATION

To begin, invoke the ether element; see the box on page 135. Then settle into a comfortable seated or reclined position and close your eyes. Visualize an oval, inside of which is a total void, in the area from your eyebrows to the crown of your head. The oval may be black or many multicolored dots. Silently repeat the mantra of ether, *ham*. Continue this practice for one to twenty minutes.

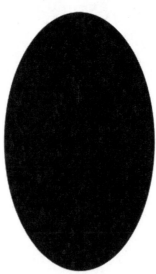

Sacred Geometry Meditation

Another simple meditation for activating the tattvas is to gaze softly at the yantra, or shape, associated with the tattva you want to invoke.

You can draw or print out the shape. (In my own product line from Divine Archetypes, the yantras are printed right on the labels of the tattva essential oil bottles. See also the color plate of the five elemental yantras at the beginning of this book.)

Gaze upon the shape for thirty to sixty seconds, trying not to blink. Then close your eyes to observe the transposition of the colors to the inside of your eyelids. Try to mentally hold and trace the sacred geometry with your mind's eye. Over time, this practice will allow you to conjure and hold these shapes in your mind's eye at will.

You can also use sacred geometry meditation to reinforce a dynamic relationship with an essential oil. For example, kaffir lime leaf essential oil holds the energy of air with the seed of fire. Its sacred geometry—a green circle with a red triangle inside—is a visual representation of this energy. You can meditate on that geometric image and know with confidence that this act conjures the entirety of kaffir lime leaf's signature and fills your entire being with its vibration and associated qualities.

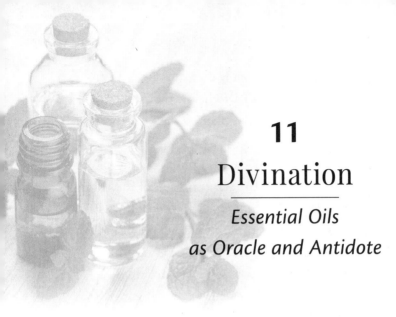

11

Divination

Essential Oils as Oracle and Antidote

Just like oracle cards or runes, essential oils are an effective divination tool. Each oracle card and rune has a specific meaning; so does each essential oil. When you allow an essential oil's energy to guide you in choosing it as a healing vibrational tool, it is sending you a message about your needs, your own hidden energies, and your path in life.

In this chapter, we'll talk about choosing essential oils energetically—that is, using them as an oracle. Once you have selected an essential oil, revisit its profile in chapter 6—or do your own research—to decode the message it's sending you. If you pick more than one oil, read their energy like a sentence and not separate topics. Take a bit of time to delve into how the oils' energies combine and what that merger means to you, in your current circumstance.

A unique aspect of using essential oils for divination is that not only do they alert you to the influence of energy patterns in your life, but they provide the specific energy you need—that is, the antidote. If you need amplification, a shift, healing, or rebalancing of an energetic complex, the oil will offer powerful support.

Oracle: Energetically Choosing Essential Oils

One of the most efficient ways to identify which energies would be of most benefit at a given time is to arrange your essential oil bottles and/or misters together and run your hand over the tops, holding the intent that the ones you need to work with will present themselves to you. Simply scan for which bottle and/or mister feels "most active." The feeling is different for all people. I generally feel active energy as cold and tingly, but it does vary, including where I feel it. Sometimes I feel it in a specific finger (this tells me that I need to invoke the energy associated with that finger in my ritual; see chapter 15 for details). Sometimes the feeling is a low, deep ache in my arm (this tells me that I have hit upon a deep causation pattern), and sometimes it is a sharp-hot energy (which indicates that the energy I need to address is new in my field, and if I address it posthaste, it will not have a chance to become a pattern). Sometimes, as my hand floats over a specific essential oil, a certain aspect of its signature will come to mind, letting me know that I should focus my intent on that aspect while working with that essential oil. My daughter mostly feels heat. Many people insist that they feel nothing yet always seem to choose what is best for them. Simply trust in the process of "feeling," whatever that means for you, for whichever energy would be most beneficial for your growth path right now.

The method of selecting essential oils just described is essentially a divination tool. By choosing what combination will best support you, you have identified energetic patterns that you need to address at that moment or that you will need to address in the near future. Thus prepared, you can move forward with focused intent and better respond to the energies you encounter along the way.

Antidote:
Directing Healing Energy

After energetically choosing an essential oil or a mister made with one, read over the profile of that oil—or do your research if you're working with an essential oil not profiled in this book—so that you better understand the energy that is presenting itself for you. If time allows, perform a ritual to direct that raw energy to the outcome that would best serve your growth path. For example, this morning I energetically picked kaffir lime leaf essential oil. Although she holds many gifts, after reading over her profile, I focused the energy on what I needed support with today: the vibration of fire organizing air, supporting the mental organization of my basic knowledge of this topic into precise content relevant to this section, while stimulating fresh insight. I chose to do ritual anointing of my third chakra (manipura), which rules the mental body and precision and refinement of thought, with the kaffir lime leaf oil. I spoke kaffir lime leaf's sacred syllables (*yam ram*), gazed upon her yantra for thirty seconds, and deeply inhaled her scent. Focusing my mind, I asked for the gifts of kaffir lime leaf's key vibrations to step forward and organize my energy.

> **Key Vibrations:**
> *Gifts*: helps you to become technique oriented and to delight in the details of working toward practical ends; gives rise to the energy of the specialist, which allows you to establish order and transform your environment by formulating your findings in a technical manner; allows you to determine which tool would be best utilized in a certain environment.
>
> *Balancing*: allows you to take information/data and create a repeatable process; aids in understanding the environment of self.

Then I thanked the energies involved and went to work. The whole process took about five minutes. Using these tools need not be difficult or lengthy; they are designed to be of service at all times, supporting all schedules. Misters offer an even more efficient practice.

Divination and Deeper Patterns

The above example demonstrates a simple daily practice to support your energetic needs as they arise. The same principles apply to developing an ongoing practice to address deeper energetic patterns. Acting as an oracle, the oils that present themselves may reveal "disturbed energy" that is present in the deep layers of the self and how to facilitate change through resonance. Following is an example of how this information, combined with information from the unconscious provided in dreams, can bring to light otherwise inaccessible energetic patterns and inform your healing practice.

Years ago, over the span of several months, essential oils and vibrational essences that address healing discordant anger consistently presented themselves to me in my personal energy work. Anger is not a dominant outward manifestation for me, and energies addressing the healing of anger had never been a pattern for me, but those essential oils and essences kept appearing day after day. Finally, after a routine doctor's appointment, I was diagnosed with a precancerous condition in my cervix—a physical manifestation of this angry energy in a very feminine part of my self.

To support my physical healing, I commissioned a healing thangka (a sacred painting) from Jampa Gyaltsen, a living master in the art of thangka painting. As a part of the ritual of creating the thangka, Jampa presented my birth date to a highly realized lama who has the sight to see which archetype from the Tibetan Buddhist pantheon is the antidote for a person's disturbed energy. The Rinpoche proclaimed that the root cause of my diseased physical manifestation was "a mind"—the same energetic pattern to which my essential oils an tional essences had alerted me!

I have long been aware of causes of discordant energy and anger in my life. One powerful source was my upbringing in a Mormon family and my feeling from a very young age that my birthright as a female was not honored. Identifying and changing those circumstances, with firm resolve to shift the dynamic, was not sufficient to overcome the psychic inertia that kept me ensnared in this anger energy. The question then became clear: What steps do I need to take to overcome this deeply embedded cultural energy that continues to trouble me? At the same time, how can I reconcile the fact that my parents actively choose that paradigm as a fostering energy for themselves?

My perspective shifted from antagonistic energy ("You did this to me, and I don't like it") to understanding that what my deep self craves and what my parents' deep selves require are vastly different. Our relationship is no longer about making them "understand me" or changing their behavior. Instead, I focus on understanding our differences with compassion and healing my angry energy around that situation. For me, this experience reinforced an important tenet: the mutability of object reality. My idea of good is very different from my parents' idea of good. Our perceptions differ based on birth karma, or elemental arrangements (see chapter 9).

Divination and Dream Work

I once had a dream that I had metal yantras of the Five Great Elements, and they were underneath my Chinese curio cabinet. When I reached under to fish out the yantras, I picked up the earth one, a square representing DNA and familial lineage healing. I started pounding on it with a round mallet with all my might. A wise man appeared; he said that I was not strong enough to break that yantra, no matter how hard I pounded. He told me to look at the shape my pounding had left on the earth yantra—a circle, which is the archetypal shape of the air element, the energy of the heart center, forgiveness, understanding, and love. He told me that what I was seeking was expressed within that sacred form and that this energy would heal my condition. The message given to me was that the anger and resentment I held for my childhood community could never be productive; that energy was not strong enough medicine to break the energetic bonds that limited me.

I used this information to craft a healing practice. I began using earth and air misters together. I anointed myself with kaffir lime leaf essential oil (air/fourth chakra) to free me from self-limiting behaviors and with galangal essential oil (earth/first chakra) for taking me deeply into family lineage healing, ultimately allowing me to attain peace and freedom from that situation.

My dreams kept me abreast of the inner work that was going on until I knew it was time to shift my tools. Many people who have used essential oils and other vibrational tools for healing have found that their dreams offer them deep insight from their unconscious, with very specific information about self, the situation, and the antidote to be used. Because our energetic continuum carries information from the evolving collective unconscious, it is very possible to wrestle internally with energy that your external self/mind has no awareness of, having no memory of the experience that caused it. You may not be able to label or even understand the root cause of this disharmonic energy, but you can employ tools that provide a healing path.

12

Formulations

Creating Targeted Essential Oil Blends

Though it's fine to use essential oils singly, it's also fun—and effective—to combine them in blends targeting different aspects of tattva, chakral, or archetypal energies. I'll give you some of my favorite formulas here, but these are just basic outlines. Please have fun playing with different base oils and essential oils that smell and feel good to you. Remember that scent is entirely subjective; if you do not enjoy one of the scent profiles, play with which essential oils you use and the number of drops until you figure out what smells and feels pleasurable to you! Just keep in mind the general ratios of essential oils and base oils for the different types of applications; see chapter 7 for more details. The formulas in this chapter call for ratios that are suitable for localized application. For full-body application, use half the amount of essential oils.

Use amber, green, blue, frosted white, or black-violet glass bottles for holding your blends. After you have added all the essential and base oils to the bottle, cap your creation and give it a gentle shake to combine all the ingredients. Shake again before each use.

Formulas to Stimulate the Chakras

While a single essential oil can be an effective way to work with a specific aspect of a chakra, a blend of essential oils allows you to address the chakra in its entirety.

Root Chakra

10 ml corn oil

12 drops patchouli essential oil

6 drops red spikenard essential oil

5 drops vetiver essential oil

Sacral Chakra

10 ml avocado oil

12 drops blood orange essential oil

4 drops vanilla essential oil

3 drops pink pepper seed essential oil

Solar Plexus Chakra

10 ml coconut oil

11 drops lemon essential oil

8 drops elemi essential oil

4 drops cardamom essential oil

3 drops black pepper essential oil

Heart Chakra

5 ml sweet almond oil

5 ml apricot kernel oil

12 drops pine essential oil

12 drops rosewood essential oil

2 drops neroli essential oil

Throat Chakra

10 ml apricot kernel oil

12 drops lavender essential oil

8 drops frankincense essential oil

2 drops blue chamomile essential oil

Third Eye Chakra

10 ml corn oil

12 drops lemon essential oil

8 drops sandalwood essential oil

2 drops jasmine essential oil

Crown Chakra

10 ml sweet almond oil

6 drops lime essential oil

4 drops rose essential oil

3 drops Chinese rice flower essential oil

1 drop white lotus essential oil

Converting Blends to Misters

Combine the essential oils from any of the blends in this chapter, in the same ratios, in a mister bottle, omitting the base oil. (Because misting is not a topical application, you can add as much essential oil as you want to create the scent profile you desire.) Add 1 teaspoon of witch hazel and fill to near the top with pure water. Gently shake to mix the ingredients.

Blends for the Nature Archetypes

Here we will explore how to energetically weave archetypes using the vibrational signatures of the essential oils we have profiled. This is a very easy skill to adapt to any archetype with which you are working. Your essential oil collection is your "thread" and comparable to using different types and colors: each string has unique qualities, and you weave them together on your loom to create a pattern. We are doing the same thing. Once you have identified the properties of each essential oil in your toolbox, you can blend the oils to create the energetic structure of any archetype. This provides a tangible medium for you to work with.

To sum up:

1. Identify the traits of the archetype you would like to work with.
2. Select the essential oils that express the same traits.
3. Blend the essential oils to create the energetic structure with which you want to work.

This is a very powerful way to honor the archetype and to make its subtle energy manifest in your life.

Goddess of the Marshlands

$1/8$ ounce apricot kernel oil

11 drops lemon essential oil

6 drops frankincense essential oil

5 drops patchouli essential oil

1 drop betel leaf essential oil

Goddess of the Moors

$1/8$ ounce corn oil

14 drops blood orange essential oil

6 drops cardamom essential oil

3 drops neroli essential oil

Acorn Dryad

$^1/_8$ ounce corn oil

8 drops vetiver essential oil

3 drops galangal essential oil

1 drop white lotus essential oil

Oak Dryad

$^1/_8$ ounce coconut oil

10 drops elemi essential oil

5 drops patchouli essential oil

1 drop blue chamomile essential oil

Weeping Willow Dryad

$^1/_8$ ounce avocado oil

15 drops lavender essential oil

6 drops pine essential oil

3 drops lime essential oil

Crocus Fairy

$^1/_8$ ounce avocado oil

5 drops rose essential oil

2 drops red spikenard essential oil

2 drops vanilla essential oil

Dogwood Fairy

$^1/_8$ ounce apricot oil

8 drops Chinese rice flower essential oil

2 drops jasmine essential oil

1 drop massoia bark essential oil

Morning Glory Fairy

$^1/_8$ ounce apricot kernel oil

14 drops rosewood essential oil

3 drops galangal essential oil

1 drop agarwood essential oil

Sunflower Fay

$^1/_8$ ounce sweet almond oil

9 drops sandalwood essential oil

5 drops lemon essential oil

3 drops black pepper essential oil

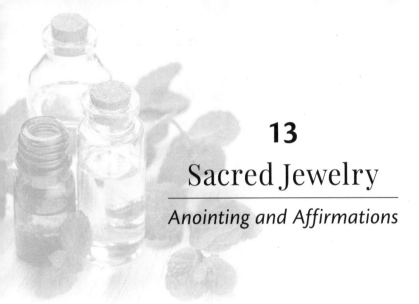

13
Sacred Jewelry
Anointing and Affirmations

While most studies in the Vedic system focus on herbal remedies, healing practices using metals and gems are an exciting aspect. Metals and gems have their own unique energetic properties, and anointing them with essential oils builds a powerful energetic synergy. Anointed sacred jewelry is a dynamic tool for stimulating, healing, opening, and working with energies in the body. The very act of preparing, anointing, and wearing a precious piece is a soothing, centering practice that supports your conscious efforts to direct your deepest aspects of the self.

Metals

Gold, silver, and copper are among the most common metals used in jewelry, and each has a different effect on the energetic body and doshas.

METAL	ENERGETIC TRAITS	EFFECT ON THE DOSHAS
Gold	Refinement, spirit, masculine energy, expression of understanding; helps you organize thoughts and act on them; hot and dry	Stabilizes vata (when used in small amounts), increases pitta, reduces kapha

METAL	ENERGETIC TRAITS	EFFECT ON THE DOSHAS
Silver	Introspection, soul, feminine energy, exploration of the unknown; rules the emotions and subconscious; cold and moist	Balances vata (when used in small amounts), reduces pitta, increases kapha
Copper	Self-awareness, beauty, alchemy; invokes balance and peacefulness	Balances all the doshas (and thus all the elements)

Gemstones

Each of the five tattvas has a related gemstone with unique qualities and energies that can aid us in our journey.

TIGER'S EYE

Tattva: Earth

Thanks to its grounding, protective, and stabilizing properties, this stone stimulates kundalini energy, encouraging it to rise in a healthful way. Tiger's eye has been used since ancient times to ward off dangerous energy, including subconscious thoughtforms, intentional black magic, and other destabilizing energies; a keynote for this stone is protection. It also collects and collates scattered energy, grounding us and providing us with sustainable energy to finish projects, ultimately allowing us to manifest our will on the physical plane. It also helps addictive personalities make changes in their routine and life.

MOONSTONE

Tattva: Water

Moonstone is not for the faint of heart—it brings to us what we need, rather than what we want! This stone is a silent "true prayer" in that it expands us beyond the childish phase of "getting what I want" and asks Spirit, "What do I need for growth?" Moonstone also helps us develop a profound emotional IQ, a relationship with the deep unconscious, and, perhaps most importantly, a connection to the energy of the divine feminine. It delivers profound teaching dreams, opens us to the flow of life and synchronistic events, and softens hard edges.

RED CARNELIAN

Tattva: Fire

This stone ushers in the energy of vitality, strength, and motivation. Red carnelian is wonderful for increasing and stabilizing analytical abilities. It helps bring clarity to our thinking process and helps us avoid or overcome fatigue. This stone also protects us from anger, resentment, and many other fire-based imbalances, whether they originate internally or externally, ultimately allowing us to transmute this energy into empathy for the human condition. This stone thaws "frozen" states of being, supporting an expressive, emotional, and sensual nature.

AMAZONITE

Tattva: Air

Amazonite heals and opens the heart. It filters the information we take in, allowing us to separate the wheat from the chaff and absorb into our subtle body only that which is wholesome. It allows us to hold opposing points of view simultaneously, without judgment, until we reach a conclusion. In general, this stone is soothing and helps clear past traumas that affect the heart.

LAPIS LAZULI

Tattva: Ether

The energy of lapis lazuli stimulates the awakening of spiritual gifts and connection to the divine. It teaches us to use the spoken word wisely and promotes the clearing of energetic-based disturbances that have manifested due to using words unwisely in the past or not speaking our truth. Ultimately this stone helps us contact and tune in to our inner muse and express this infinitely creative aspect of the self. This stone is also constantly at work refining our grosser aspects and gently supporting us in moving toward an enlightened state.

Imbuing Jewelry with Healing Intent

Creating a healing practice around sacred jewelry is rather straightforward. While wearing jewelry on its own offers energetic benefits, those energies can be greatly amplified by anointment with appropriate essential oils and using an affirmation to set your intent.

ANOINTMENT

You can anoint jewelry (or any other healing tool, for that matter) with essential oils or a mister made from them. If you're using an essential oil, you will generally dilute it in a base oil, using about one drop of essential oil per tablespoon of base oil. For both oils, choose ones with the desired energetic properties (see chapters 7 and 8). Pour the base oil into a small, ritually consecrated bowl.* Add the essential oil. Mix with the finger whose signature resonates with the energy you are invoking (see chapter 15). Which hand you use depends on your intent. Your right hand has the same energy as silver, while your left hand has the same energy as gold. To amplify gold's energy, mix the blend and anoint your piece with your right hand. To amplify silver's energy, use your left hand. Because copper balances all the doshas, use whichever hand carries the energy you are invoking (see pages 172–73). Anoint your jewelry piece with the oil mixture as you recite a personal affirmation for the energy you are asking to work with or review the oil's properties. When you are finished, gently buff your piece to a shine with a clean, soft cloth.

If you're using a mister, simply spray it over your jewelry piece and

---

*This is optional, but if you desire to do so, wash your bowl in salted water, rinse with fresh water, and dry with a white cloth. This will remove any energy that the bowl might hold from the store where it was purchased, a previous owner, or previous uses, creating a pristine space for the intent of your ritual.

then gently buff the piece with a clean, soft cloth, reciting your affirmation as you work.

AFFIRMATIONS

An essential aspect of vibrational healing and spiritual growth is to connect to and be present with the energy you are working with in the moment. Affirmations are a practical, concrete way of making this connection. They help us focus our intent and invoke the energetic aspect with which we seek to work.

As an example, when I am working with fire and ether, I might turn to a necklace of gold and lapis lazuli as a helpful vibrational tool. To amplify the necklace's energetic effects, I could anoint it with one drop of galangal essential oil in a teaspoon of coconut oil. Coconut oil as the base provides the stabilizing energy that fire and ether need to birth a new idea into the physical plane. Galangal offers the archetype of Lakshmi, the goddess of good fortune, and brings the energy of achieving goals, fulfilling your potential through wise action, and aligning with beneficial circumstances. As I anoint the necklace with this blend, I might say, "Please help me cultivate focused, inspired thought for my project, Lakshmi. Your grace is like the full-blooming lotus. Please endow me with your attributes and blessings. Shower abundance on all levels into my life, and bring this light by the ripening of my talents and understanding of the correct expression of my gifts. Thank you." I could then wear my necklace with the conviction that my internal elements are organizing themselves to perfectly support the invoked energy pattern of fire, ether, coconut, and Lakshmi.

Dynamic Pairings

Of course, there are many ways to combine the energies of metals, gems, anointing oils, and affirmations to craft sacred jewelry as unique vibrational tools for your own personal practice. Following are a few suggestions.

MATCHING ENERGIES FOR AMPLIFICATION

You can match element (metal and gem) to element (essential oil) to amplify a specific energy with which you want to work. For example, if you want to invoke water energy to work with your emotional body, you could pair a silver moonstone piece with agarwood essential oil, because both stimulate water. This amplification of pairing a gem and essential oil that vibrate to the same element provides a nurturing way to access your emotions.

BLENDING ENERGIES

You can mix different elements to bring about a desired effect. Remember that each essential oil and gem/metal has its own specific signature (vibrational pattern) in addition to its elemental arrangement. For example, you might anoint a silver and lapis lazuli piece, which together hold the energy of a portal into the deep mysteries/void, with massoia bark essential oil (earth/water/air) with the specific intent to utilize the plant's vibrational pattern of being a dynamic catalyst for peeling back the layers of the false self. You could use this jewelry-essence pairing in meditations that require more than the logical mind, such as when you meditate on the koan, asking, "What is my original face?"

REDIRECTING EXCESSIVE ENERGY

If you are saturated with too much of a specific element, you can redirect the energy. For example, if you have too much earth energy, you might feel stuck and stagnant. To move this energy, you would first access muladhara, the first chakra, which is linked to the earth element, and stimulate it with a vibrational tool that can reduce the earth energy, like a copper jewelry piece (copper balances all the elements). Then you might anoint yourself or an amulet you'll wear with an essential oil featuring fire, water, air, or ether to promote movement in the desired direction. If you want to foster creativity, comprehension, or dynamic action, for example, over the stagnation of excessive earth energy, you could select an essential oil or mister that supports that pattern.

BALANCING ENERGIES TO CULTIVATE HARMONY

You can also use essential oils to balance the specific energy of the metal from which the jewelry piece is made. A balancing approach can be particularly useful if a piece of jewelry's energy is not in complete harmony with your body type. For example, silver's energy is cold and moist; vata is also cold, but dry. If a dominant vata type wants to wear a silver amulet for exploration of subconscious emotional patterns (silver rules emotions and the subconscious), the cold of the metal could become aggravating. To offset this effect, you could anoint the silver amulet with an essential oil featuring the fire element, which brings heat.

14
Mantras and Yantras
Amplification Practices

The proper usage of a plant or herb, during which its true power is released, implies a communion with it. . . . This means giving value to a plant as something sacred, as a means of communion with all nature. Each plant, then, like a mantra, will help to actualize the potential of cosmic life of which it is a representative. . . .

Yantras can also be used to . . . potentize (increase the power and depth of penetration) medicines, as well as to purify the treatment room. They can be placed on certain parts of the body, like the chakras, to release blockages. In this regard they can be used in conjunction with crystals and gem-stones.

DAVID FRAWLEY, *THE YOGA OF HERBS*

We can support plants' healing powers and potentize essential oils through the use of sacred sounds and symbols during the preparation and application of the oils. Because the realm of sounds and symbols is vast, here we will explore only those specifically related to the tattvas.

In various Eastern traditions, sacred sounds and symbols are known, respectively, as *mantras* and *yantras*.

What Are Mantras and Yantras?

Mantra is a Sanskrit word that can be translated literally as "instrument of thought." More loosely, a mantra is a sacred sound, word, or group of words with healing or transformational capabilities. In the context of using essential oils, mantras may be used as instruments for directing the healing and transformational energies of the plants (from which the oils are derived) into the mind. According to Vedic scholar David Frawley, "The mind is refined through plants. In the *mantra* it is perfected. . . . [The mantra] gives herbs a power of psychological healing and spiritual integration. It brings the universal intelligence of nature into harmony with the individual."[1]

Without right intent, the healing process remains superficial. Use of a mantra makes the healing process a conscious act. But repetition of a mantra must itself be a conscious act, not merely a mechanical one. Right use of a mantra is an act of meditation for penetration into and manifestation of the inner truth—a means of healing consciousness. Consciously performing a mantra while preparing an essential oil blend, or while applying the blend (either to yourself or, if you are a hands-on healer, to a client or patient), will greatly increase the potency of the oils.

The visual counterpart to a mantra is a yantra. *Yantra* is also a Sanskrit word, and its meaning is contextual. Whereas a mantra is a creative vibration, a yantra can be taken as the pattern created by that vibration. A yantra can be a symbol that represents the quintessential nature of a concept, helping the mind focus on and grasp the concept. Such a symbol can be a geometric shape as simple as a circle or square, or it can be as complex as a mandala.

Yantras come in many forms. They may be drawn, painted, sewn, or sculpted using various media, such as paper, fabric, wood, stone, or metal, and they can be used in many ways. Healing preparations (e.g., essential oil blends) may be created with, or in the presence of, one or more yantras, so as to potentize such preparations. Yantras may be displayed or used in a healing space to purify it or placed on the chakras to release blockages. "*Yantras* . . . serve to draw in the cosmic life force and establish a space for healing to occur. With the *mantra,* they purify the astral aura and cleanse the psychic environment, which is always impure or stagnant in the case of disease."[2]

Many Eastern traditions believe that the mental continuum (or, loosely, the mind) has the greatest influence on our well-being. Consequently, "training" the mind by introducing wholesome vibrations can literally reshape the energetic body, which will in turn affect the physical and emotional bodies, allowing us to move toward a state of wholeness. We can produce desirable vibrations by repeating specific mantras (aloud or silently) and focusing our gaze on specific yantras with meditative and therapeutic intent.

Some methodologies purport that you must repeat a mantra 100,000 times before its energy is fully empowered, but even a single utterance of a mantra can bring benefit. The *Rig Veda* reads like a how-to manual for using magic sounds and incantations to shape reality, addressing everything from asking plants for assistance in a healing process to getting rid of a rival wife. In my current healing practice, a significant aspect of my work is silently repeating an appropriate mantra to help me consciously connect with the plants I use in my blends, while laying warmed large pink onyx yantras of the Five Great Elements on the corresponding chakras to powerfully support the plants' healing powers during a treatment.

Some Fundamental Mantras and Yantras

Here the focus is on a select few mantras and yantras relevant to our study of the tattvas. The following table shows the mantras and yantras associated with the elements, along with the corresponding chakras whose energies arise from the elements.

MANTRA	YANTRA	ELEMENT	CHAKRA
Ham	Black oval	Ether	Fifth (throat)
Yam	Smoky-green circle	Air	Fourth (heart)
Ram	Red triangle (pointing upward)	Fire	Third (navel)
Vam	Silver crescent moon	Water	Second (sacral)
Lam	Yellow square	Earth	First (root)

In addition to the elemental mantras, there are two more mantras described by Frawley as prime mantras.

OM: the most important of all mantras, it represents the Divine Word itself. It serves to energize or empower all things and all processes. Therefore all mantras begin and end with OM. OM clears the mind, opens the channels and increases Ojas [water on a vital level]. It is the sound of affirmation that allows us to accept who we are and open up to the positive forces of the universe. OM is the sound of Prana and the sound of the inner light that takes our energy up the spine. It awakens the positive life-force (Prana) necessary for healing to occur. It opens up all the potential of consciousness. . . .

HUM (pronounced with the "u" sound as in our word "put"): an excellent mantra for warding off negative influences attacking us, whether disease-causing pathogens, negative emotions, or even black magic. It is also the best mantra for awakening Agni, either as the digestive fire or the fire of the mind. It is good for burning up toxins, whether physically or psychologically, and for cleansing the channels. It increases Tejas [fire on a vital level] and the perceptive powers of the mind (Buddhi) and gives control over our desire nature. It is sacred to Shiva, the God of transformation, and is the sound of Divine wrath.[3]

Frawley's pronouncement that *om* begins and ends all mantras requires some clarification. Obviously, because mantras can be single syllables or words, his statement is not strictly true. However, many multi-word mantras do begin with *om* but don't necessarily end with it. Instead, *om* is often used at the end of a meditation in which a mantra may be repeated many times, rather than at the end of every repetition of the mantra.

One well-known mantra that begins with *om* and ends with *hum* is the Buddhist mantra *om mani padme hum*. It is the mantra of Avalokiteshvara, the Buddha of compassion. While this mantra cannot be directly translated into sensible English, it is said to contain the essence of all the teachings of the Buddha, and saying it (or even viewing the written form, as a yantra) is said to invoke the great compassion of Avalokiteshvara.

Tyler Dewar describes *om* and *hum* as follows:

The white OM . . . is the syllable of combined qualities and is of the nature of the perfection of meditation. It purifies the mental affliction of pride, along with all the results thereby produced. . . .

The black HUM . . . is the syllable of mind and is of the nature of the perfection of supreme knowledge. It purifies dualistic anger, along with all the results thereby produced.[4]

Finally, there is the mantra *svaha,* or *soha*. This one is not typically used alone but rather at the end of a multi-word mantra. It may be translated as "May this come about." It indicates our desire to plant the root of the path to enlightenment in our hearts. More generally, it may be used to reinforce our intent to achieve our highest state of well-being and wholeness of mind and body.

Constructing a Personal Mantra

Now let's explore some simple ways to construct a multi-word mantra from the single-word mantras described above to achieve "right conditioning" (or a properly balanced state) of mind and body. We'll start with *om*, then choose one or more elemental mantras (from the table above), and end with *hum, soha,* or both. The possible combinations look like this:

OM + elemental mantra(s) + HUM
OM + elemental mantra(s) + SOHA
OM + elemental mantra(s) + HUM + SOHA

In constructing a mantra, you should take into account not only the tattva with which you seek to work but also your primary dosha. As a very simple guide, those who are primarily vata should use mantras that are warm and calming; pitta types should use mantras that are cool and calming; and kapha types should use mantras that are warm and stimulating.

Mantras that are beneficial for ether/air types (vata):

+ *Ram* (fire) brings warmth, protection, focus, and direction.
+ *Lam* (earth) brings stabilization and grounding.
+ *Vam* (water) is soothing and calming to vatas' sometimes frantic and frazzled natures.

Mantras that are beneficial for fire types (pitta):

+ *Ham* (ether) is cooling; it helps fire types escape from the bounds of ego and reach up toward their higher natures.
+ *Vam* (water) cools hot emotions; it assists us in becoming free from the constraints of the mind and opening to positive emotions and the soul body.
+ *Yam* (air) opens the heart.

Mantras that are beneficial for water/earth types (kapha):

+ *Ham* (ether) awakens the connection to our celestial roots, breathing the divine back into kaphas' sometimes pragmatic forms.
+ *Yam* (air) fosters forgiveness (kapha types are more likely to hold grudges than other types).
+ *Ram* (fire) incites motion, ambition, and the passion to get things done.

People generally repeat mantras aloud, but doing so for more than a short period of time may be taxing for vata, so you may wish to switch to silent chanting after some chanting aloud. Keep in mind that chanting aloud does not necessarily mean forceful chanting. Chanting can be soft and gentle. Of course, as you go about your daily activities in public, you may wish to always chant silently, regardless of your dosha.

Creating a Potentizing Practice

Incorporating your knowledge of the elemental and chakral properties (see chapters 3 and 4), you can effectively integrate mantras and yantras into your practice. Your practice can be as simple or as elaborate as you like. As a very simple example, one of my clients recently told me that, in an effort to channel the gifts of earth energy into her day, she had taken to drawing golden squares (the earth yantra) on the soles of her shoes and anointing her socks with galangal essential oil (which carries earth energy) while repeating *lam* (the earth mantra).

As an example of a more elaborate practice, I incorporated mantra and yantra work into my practice for healing discordant anger arising from familial/DNA patterns (which I uncovered through dream work and energetic essential oil selection). To create the oil blend that I used for anointing my amulets and chakras, I combined 1 tablespoon of apricot kernel oil, 2 drops of kaffir lime leaf essential oil, and 3 drops of galangal essential oil. I blended the oils in a small bowl using the middle finger of my left hand (which holds the energy of dealing with difficulties head-on and releasing them), and I repeated the mantra *om lam vam hum* over the mixture eleven times (eleven is the vibration of disconnecting from the collective; see chapter 16). I applied the blend to my earth center (first chakra), tracing a square, and then to my air center (fourth chakra), tracing a circle. After anointing myself, I laid my hands on those chakras while reclining in meditation, repeating the given mantra 108 times. Additionally, each day I wore a specific necklace—one with a copper square and a silver circle and anointed with the same blend I used for anointing the chakras—to reinforce the healing vibration I had introduced into my field.

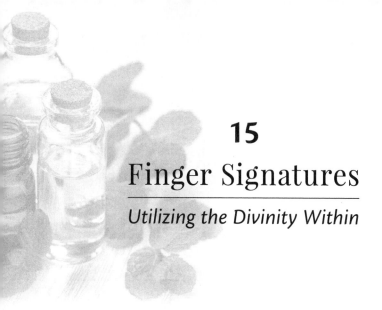

15
Finger Signatures

Utilizing the Divinity Within

In studying finger signatures, we invoke the principle of microcosm and macrocosm, remembering that the energy we invoke for healing is not "out there somewhere" but inside us. Various parts of the physical human body, including the hands, hold the energy of specific archetypes. When we use a particular finger to mix our blends, we summon all of the archetypal energies associated with that finger, including deity, gem, planet, and element aspects of the self, and we instill the qualities associated with those energies into the blend. This practice helps us experiment more consciously with various emanations of the divine within and allows us to see the effects of the resonant vibration in the outer world on self and environment.

There is wide variance between schools of thought regarding the study and interpretation of the following associations. For example, many schools expound that Saturn is a negative energy, but I most emphatically disagree. I feel that Saturn is our inner parent. The chart on the following page provides a snapshot of my interpretation of several Eastern and Western schools of thought combined. Below the chart is further information on the vibrational/energetic patterns of these five aspects (digit, element, planet, gem, and deity) and how they relate to one another.

DIGIT	ELEMENT	PLANET	GEM	DEITY
Pointer (index) finger	Air	Jupiter	Yellow sapphire	Zeus
Middle finger	Fire	Saturn	Blue sapphire	Saturn/ Cronus
Ring finger	Water	Sun	Ruby	Apollo
Pinky finger	Earth	Mercury	Emerald	Hermes
Thumb	Ether	Venus	Diamond	Aphrodite/ Inanna/ Ishtar

Breaking It Down

Let's take a look at some of the ways in which the qualities of each finger signature mesh with the qualities of the energetic aspects with which it is associated.

Pointer Finger

Qualities: Authority, charisma, and leadership

Air: New thought, sudden insights, and breakthroughs

Jupiter: Philosophy, expansion, higher thought, and abundance

Yellow sapphire: Attracts affluence and expands the intellect so we see the big picture

Zeus: Regality, authority, and taking care of and protecting those in need

Middle Finger

Qualities: Creating structure, boundaries, and organization

Fire: Good comprehension, liveliness, awareness, and enthusiasm

Saturn: Using hard work to solve problems and having strength to deal head-on with difficulties

Blue sapphire: Tranquillity, staying on a spiritual path, and transmuting negative energies

Saturn/Cronus: Working with all shadow issues, understanding time, and working with setbacks and limitations

Ring Finger

Qualities: Artistic expansion through established channels, emotional distance, moderation, and bringing chaos into order

Water: Imagination and accessing the subconscious and emotions

Sun: Masculine energy, refinement, brilliance, and being conscious

Ruby: Energy, vitality, and enthusiasm for life (may overstimulate those who are particularly sensitive)

Apollo: To "know thyself" and to promote "nothing in excess"; helpful for learning a classical art (language, painting, sculpting, music, etc.) in a recognized style

Pinky Finger

Qualities: Traveling between dimensions, communication, making choices swiftly, and acting quickly

Earth: Being supportive/supported, grounded, and nurturing; accumulation

Mercury: Dream work, active imagination, success in public speaking or business, and receiving esoteric messages

Emerald: Helps us operate in the "As above, so below" paradigm, heals the heart, promotes mental clarity and balance, raises consciousness

Hermes: God of alchemy, good luck, the unexpected, coincidences, and synchronicity; opens us to gaiety, joy, ingenuity, nature spirits, and working with our inner psychopomp (soul guide)

Thumb

Qualities: Passionate love, sensuality, sexual-spiritual force, sex appeal, primal force of nature, muse energy, and the animating vital force that dwells in all matter

Ether: Expansion, no limitations, the unknown, the dry void, and information beyond the rational

Venus: Wild abandon, unregulated artistry, appreciation for beauty, enjoying sensual pleasures (i.e., wine, fragrant massage, food, scented baths), learning through the senses

Diamond: Bonding love relationships, attracting abundance, bringing about transformation by shining a light on disharmonious patterns, and stimulating spiritual understanding

Aphrodite/Inanna/Ishtar: This goddess archetype is the morning and night star, meaning she embodies both the dark and bright goddess energies; considered alchemical and unpredictable, neither easy to regulate nor for the faint of heart

Invoking Finger Signatures

Because each digit manifests myriad energies, establishing intent is essential. If you wish to invoke only a partial vibration, simply hold your intent to activate that particular energy as you mix your essential oil blend. If you want to enliven the entire spectrum of energy, keep that intent in mind as you work.

The general rule is to use the left hand to invoke feminine energy and the right to call in masculine energy.

Using the left hand invokes the feminine traits of:

+ Lunar energy and all that it holds
+ Intuition and knowing beyond the gross mind
+ Traversing into the unknown, including the subconscious mind
+ Undoing gently
+ Stillness and receiving

+ Patience
+ Nurturing, fostering, and embryonic forms
+ The mystical

Using the right hand invokes the masculine traits of:

+ Solar energy and all that it holds
+ Synthesis and refinement of deep mystery for conscious use
+ Strong intellect, being conscious, and superior analytical traits
+ Force
+ Dynamic action
+ Protection
+ Joy, laughter, and warmth
+ Virility and potency

16

Numerological Signatures

Measurements as Vibrations

As with finger signatures, there are many different approaches to numerology. The chart below lists my interpretation of the vibration of numbers 1 through 13. (All numbers have vibrations, but 1 through 13 seems like a reasonably sized toolbox, and those are the numbers I use in my own practice.) Keep in mind that this is just a snapshot; the listed qualities comprise only part of each number's signature, and there is much more to the overall pattern.

NUMBER	QUALITIES
1	Unity, all that is, undivided universal energy, the alchemical marriage, and wholeness
2	Polarity, that which divides, male and female energies, and duality
3	The Trinity, the undivided primal waters, the Sophia wisdom energy, and the Logos energy operating in each individual*
4	Foundation, practicality, structure, and order
5	Understanding inner divinity, micro- and macrocosm associations, and loving the human experience
6	Structured dynamism, the ability to spontaneously respond to the moment, and allowing that feedback to restructure the self
7	Mystical understanding, universal truths, and how we can best use this understanding for the highest good of all

NUMBER	QUALITIES
8	Earthly power, acquisition, navigating practical circumstances, strength, being firm, and time versus eternity
9	Greater cycles of expansion, self-mastery, access to the emotional body, humanitarian acts, love given and received, and opening to our inner genius
10	Manifestation through clear intentions and connection to the collective†
11	Dissolution of form, intuition, pulling apart limitations to release new potential, and disconnecting from the collective
12	Stability in movement and the ability to radically expand while staying centered in our self without disorientation
13	Wild unseen forces, synchronicity, asking for divine direction, working with oracles, and opening to the unknown

*The *undivided primal waters* are pure potentiality, the "all thing" before taking form. *Sophia* is gnosis, or knowledge so great that it cannot be caged by the average human mind and is more felt and understood in an amorphous way. This energy is sometimes described as the "fire" of knowing or a testimony to a truth that cannot be proved or even articulated but is so powerful that it shapes lives and destinies. *Logos* can be understood as the expression of divine archetypal energy that has dropped into form at a dense enough vibration that the human mind can begin to organize, process, and utilize the divine information being expressed and act upon it.

†*Collective* can be understood in this context as the unified understanding and experience of a joint reality.

Applying Number Vibrations

You can make use of the vibrational energy of numbers in determining the number of drops of an essential oil to use in a blend. For example, four drops of an essential oil in a blend could help you undertake foundational work or the solid building of an enterprise. Seven drops would be ideal for creating a meditation blend to help open you to universal truths. Eleven drops would be helpful when disconnecting from a circumstance, such as a relationship or job that you have outgrown.

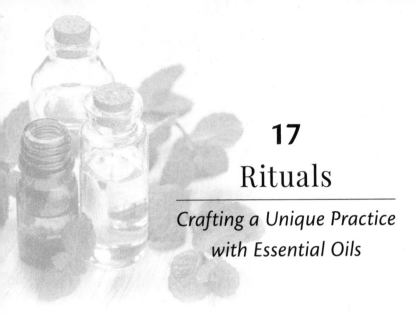

17
Rituals

Crafting a Unique Practice with Essential Oils

The essence of ritual is that something is done in the physical realm that is related to the higher worlds. This may be a simple gesture of the hand or an elaborate ceremony. It can be working consciously in everyday life, so that quite mundane actions become full of meaning, or a carefully designed ritual acted out for specific occasion. . . . Ritual is the mode of formalizing action and giving it not only meaning, but creating a contact with other worlds.

Z'EV BEN SHIMON HALEVI,
THE SCHOOL OF KABBALAH

Any affect or emotion which in its raw and unaltered form is too intense to be controlled by will alone may need its ritual.

Without ritual, such energies may inundate the ego and force it into acting out or into obsessive behavior. Ritual brings about containment and acceptance, control of intensity, and "dosage."

EDWARD WHITMONT, *THE SYMBOLIC QUEST*

One of the main obstacles that keeps us from being able to plug into archetypes and spontaneously take on unadulterated understanding is the obscuration of our pure self, which is buried beneath habituated, dense, negative energy patterns. We must clear the debris away from our own pure nature before we can easily embody archetypal patterns. We use rituals to do this work.

The first step in this process is using rituals to consciously clear space or heal emotional-mental-spiritual disturbances. There are myriad reasons for these disturbances: birth karma, emotional trauma, an unhealthy family/childhood, distorted mental understanding, or cultural conditioning, for example. Labeling the source of the energy obscuring the pure self is not as important as understanding how to address whatever unhealthy energy is present and applying the correct antidote. One of my favorite stories illuminating this point comes from the Buddha: When the Buddha was asked, "What is the source of distorted ego?" he answered, "Do you try to find out how the arrow became lodged in your eye before you remove it? Or do you just pull it out?"

This does not imply that we should not do personal work to decipher the root causes of unhealthy behaviors. That work is vital, but we must also remember to act *in the immediate* by addressing what is obvious and available to work with. As we stabilize volatile emotions and expand clear mental understanding, we gain the ability to address root causes more effectively.

One reason for working with the disturbed energy that most readily reveals itself is that often it is just the tip of the iceberg in that specific energy complex. It may indicate deeper content that is still submerged, out of reach of the conscious mind, and struggling to make itself known, understood, integrated, or healed. This ties in to the concept of "shadow possessions." When the ego refuses to examine its own dark aspects, they remain repressed in the interior layer of the personal unconscious. But all that we deny, fear, or hate in ourselves becomes projected into our environment as a teaching tool (albeit a rough one).

When the "pious" ego self denies its own depth of dark, this content is then projected onto personal, family, or cultural scapegoats. When we are overtaken by our repressed aspects, an amoral, inflated craziness (a superior sense of self) ensues. So, if you are especially triggered by a particular event, circumstance, or person, pay close attention, and immediately start to treat that energy with the corresponding essential oils and other supporting remedies.

Rituals turn us inward so that archetypes can be activated; rituals also express unconscious forces and help us through difficult transitional stages. Rituals give us a safe way to explore our own darkness. This timeless act of invoking an energy (archetypal form) much greater than what our small conscious self is capable of is usually employed when the "mind" is blocked and we cannot figure out our next steps.

Ritual is, at its most basic level, a manifestation of intent—an act or ceremony that functions as a conscious invocation of a particular energy or outcome. Intent is a powerful force on the vibrational level. As David Stewart, Ph.D., cofounder and president of the Center for Aromatherapy Research and Education, notes, it can influence the vibration of an essential oil negatively or positively. He offers the following numbers.

1. Negative thoughts lower frequencies by 12 MHz.
2. Positive thoughts raise frequencies by 10 MHz.
3. Prayer raises frequencies by 15 MHz.[1]

The astonishing vibrational effect of prayer—the focused intent of communication with the divine—highlights the importance of admixing ritual into our daily life and essential oil practice. In whatever form suits best, as massoia bark teaches us, life is alive, and we must adapt and respond from moment to moment, from day by day, to what action is needed most. Ritual gives us a conscious space in which to tune in and respond to the energies around us. As we learn to consciously create that ritual space, the entire vibration of our surroundings becomes responsive to our changing needs and is able to interact with us in a more meaningful, supportive way. Dare to live this way, reveling in the fact that all that surrounds you—people, creatures, objects, energies—is a living, breathing organism intelligently responding to you!

There are many ways to incorporate essential oils into simple rituals to enhance your spiritual development and support you on your path to your highest self. Following are some examples, but keep in mind that you can create your own rituals as you wish. A part of the fun of working with essential oils is familiarizing yourself with all of its aspects—including its associated tattvas, chakras, and archetypes—and designing rituals to support your specific needs.

Indicators of Vibrational Healing

When you are working with essential oils for vibrational healing and spiritual growth, it is very common to experience strong, disquieting emotions. These should be understood as energetic patterns rising to the surface to be consciously examined, understood, and finally transmuted. This process can feel overwhelming at times, but it is paramount to remember during a "healing crisis" that you should not abandon your practice before completing the cycle, no matter how difficult. Continue with the meditations, visualizations, mantras, affirmations, and other ritual work until the energy shifts.

If you need extra support during this journey, you will find a list of recommended healers at the end of the book who can help walk you through your personal process. *Remember, the key is to stay in process!*

Energetic reactions may include but are not limited to:

- Strong vivid dreams ripe with meaning, which may be frightening at times

- Physical manifestations of energy moving and reshaping matter
- Wild emotions and rapid, radical shifts in knowing and understanding
- Feeling more tired than normal, or feeling slightly "fuzzy" or "wobbly"
- Changes in appetite
- Needing time alone to process
- Long-forgotten memories rising to the surface
- Urgency around accomplishments and goals
- Clarity around dramatic life changes, and life opening up to support this
- The development of internal resolve to change long-standing patterns
- Feeling at peace and supported
- Ease of movement
- Building a deeper understanding of self and what this means
- Excitement at facing challenges head-on
- Feeling in control even during difficult or challenging circumstances
- Achieving unshakable internal equanimity
- Refinement of the mental, emotional, and intuitive bodies
- Compassion, grace, and understanding for humankind underscoring every action
- Profound personal and spiritual development
- Understanding which energetic tools are required for reaching specific ends

Invoking Divine Archetypal Energy with an Anointment Ritual

This ritual invokes the Dark Goddess using betel leaf and agarwood essential oils for anointment. Remember that this is just an example;

you can create your own rituals with any essential oil to invoke the associated archetypes.

Ingredients

½ ounce apricot kernel oil

11 drops agarwood essential oil

6 drops betel leaf essential oil

Apricot oil, in this case, stimulates exchange between the subtle and mental bodies, allowing you to commune more easily with the divine energies. Agarwood helps you to move past reflexive emotional states, and the number eleven brings the gift of dissolution of form, pulling apart what limits you to release new potential. Betel leaf holds the vibration of the Dark Goddess, and the number six provides structured dynamism, allowing you to spontaneously respond to the moment and allowing that feedback to restructure the self.

Blending the Oils

1. Pour the apricot base oil into a clean ½-ounce bottle (preferably dark glass), being sure to leave enough room for the essential oils.

2. If needed, liquefy the agarwood: Bring a small saucepan of water to a boil, reduce the heat to low, and set the agarwood bottle in the hot water. Let the bottle sit in the hot water until its contents become liquid.

3. Add the agarwood and betel leaf essential oils to the bottle with the apricot oil.

4. Cap the bottle. Roll it back and forth thirteen times in your hands while calling on each plant by name—apricot, agarwood, betel leaf—to come to support you and teach you the gift each holds. Thank them one by one for their help. (The number thirteen brings wild unseen forces, synchronicity, and opening to the unknown.)

Enlivening Ritual

1. Wrap the bottle in a dark cloth.

2. While gently holding your bottle, invoke the Dark Mother (or whichever of her manifestations you most resonate with, such as Kali, the Black Madonna, or Sophia) and ask her to enliven your cocktail of oils, repeating the archetypal incantation: *Mother, divine, black, and perfect, I call upon you to rip asunder all that is incorrect, to give me the strength to hold my position against all opposition, and to call to me all who will support my journey into wholeness as I birth my new way of being. Hold me in the velvet of your arms. Feed me and cradle me as I grow out of your dark perfection. Amen.*

3. Set your bottle on a windowsill overnight so that it can soak in the rich night energy.

Anointment

Apply the enlivened anointing oil to your body in the following order: the center of the sole of each foot, your belly, your heart, the back of your neck, the center of your forehead, and the crown of your head. As you start, visualize the dark, rich energy of the soil being pulled up in to your feet; feel that energy rising up through your body as you anoint, and finally being released into the universe. Finish with a dab of the oil on each wrist for smelling throughout the day. You can use anywhere from just a few drops up to a dime-size dab of oil on each spot.

Anoint yourself up to three times daily. Use this ritual to call the Dark Goddess into your life so that you can actively work with her energy.

Invoking Water Energy with a Bathing Ritual

Water represents feelings, sensitivities, inner process, and cleansing. So when you add a blend of essential oils to your bathwater and then activate it with ritual and intent, your tub is overflowing with the energy of those plants and the archetypal energy to create dynamic change. Water can also memorize, amplify, and replicate any information, infusing your body to the core with augmented healing energy. The average human body is roughly 70 percent water, so our own ability to copy, memorize, and maintain new energy is remarkable! Keep this in mind as you immerse yourself in your essential oil blend, and step out of the tub refreshed and literally a new you!

The following is a bath ritual intended to invoke increase and abundance, and to use self as the vehicle to do so. Remember, this is just an example; you may use this basic formula to work with other essential oil blends.

Ingredients

1 cup coconut milk

10 drops galangal essential oil

In this blend, the coconut milk supports perseverance in completing tasks, which in turn helps us manifest our full potential. It also provides strong, steady energy and the ability to welcome challenges and be solution oriented. We use ten drops of galangal because the number ten brings the vibration of manifestation through clear intention and connection to the collective.

Enlivening Ritual

1. If needed, liquefy the galangal: Bring a small saucepan of water to a boil, reduce the heat to low, and set the galangal bottle in the hot water. Let the bottle sit in the hot water until its contents become liquid.

2. Combine the coconut milk and galangal in a glass bowl. Mix with the thumb of your left hand (this combination brings expansion, release from limitations, artistry, and nurturing), mentally focusing on the associated attributes you are infusing into your blend.

3. Holding the bowl with both hands, speak into the bowl, repeating

the mantra for galangal, *lam vam,* until the mixture feels enlivened to you.

4. Next, speak aloud the associated archetypal incantation: *Lakshmi, your grace is like the full-blooming lotus. Please endow me with your attributes and blessings. Shower wealth into my life, and bring this light by the ripening of my talents and understanding of the correct expression of my gifts. Please open the lotus in my heart and take away the darkness of self-doubt, stagnation, fear, and procrastination. Allow every breath I take to be one of grace, enabling me to move forward in beautiful expression.*

Bathing Ritual

1. Bring the enlivened blend into your bathroom and close the door. Declare the room a sacred ritual space by turning off the electric lights and lighting the room with six white unscented candles (the number six brings the energy of structured dynamism, allowing you to respond to the moment, and allowing that feedback to restructure the self). After the candles have burned for a few minutes, add one drop of galangal essential oil to the softened wax of each. (One drop of galangal brings the energy of stability and wholeness, making you the container to hold and grow your goal.) Play some sort of beautiful music; I recommend something purely instrumental that is enchanting and uplifting, like Bach's *Air on the G String* for violin and piano.

2. Draw a bath, adding your blend to the running water as an offering. As the tub fills, ask the overlying energy pattern of galangal to come and support you in your growth; envision Lakshmi and Otter stretching your energetic blueprint, awakening their expansive energy within you. Stir the water in a figure-eight pattern, the infinity symbol (for empowerment), going over in your mind specific things you would like to foster and grow. Ask for white and tangerine light to infuse your bathwater and every cell of your body (white is the color of water itself, and tangerine the color of galangal), bringing you a

more perfect understanding of correct action and support on your journey.

3. Slide into the bathtub, asking for your energetic, emotional, and mental bodies to be fostered and guided toward understanding the correct action that you need to take next, and to be open to understanding your divine plan by recognizing and responding to synchronistic events. Then lie back in the warm water, relax, enjoy, and absorb the vibration.

4. When you are ready, let the water drain out, and visualize any limiting emotion, thought, or behavior being released and floating down the drain, gone forever.

Invoking Fire Energy with an Aromatherapy Ritual

This is a general example of a ritual utilizing a tea light diffuser, where you fill the bowl of the upper portion with water, add a few drops of essential oil, and then set a tea candle beneath it; as the flame heats the water, the essential oil vaporizes into the air, gently diffusing its aroma. You could easily use a different kind of diffuser.

Ingredients

Springwater

9 drops kaffir lime leaf essential oil

Kaffir lime leaf creates momentum around the act of doing good works. You can, of course, use a different kind of essential oil here to support a different goal.

Aromatherapy Ritual

1. Fill the bowl of an aromatherapy candle diffuser with springwater, and ask the water to amplify the gifts of the plants.

2. Add nine drops of the kaffir lime leaf to the water. (The number nine

brings the energy of greater cycles of expansion and humanitarian acts.)

3. Light the tea candle. Set your intention for the flame to connect to the spark of your soul, igniting what is divine in you, and burning away the dross (waste matter) so that you are left with only your essential self and can see clearly what is to be done next.

4. As the fragrance fills your home, breathe deeply, breathing in as you consciously own your intention and breathing out what no longer serves you.

5. Chant kaffir lime leaf's mantra, *yam ram*, at least seven times to help you align with the air and fire elements you are invoking. (The number seven helps you understand universal truths and how to best utilize this understanding for the betterment of all.)

6. Once you feel your mind settle, speak the associated archetypal incantation to help support your goal: *Tara, imbue me with the wisdom and strength to be like you, "quick like lightning" in recognizing and aiding others in need, be it hunger of spirit and soul or need on the physical level. Allow me to see the most skillful and swift means of balancing any imbalance. Help me move forward until every one of my brothers' and sisters' needs are met with the same standards I require for myself, be it the need for education, freedom of thought and expression, ample recourses, a healthy environment, or a safe, positive space that encourages growth. Bless me with the divine sensitivity not to push my understanding of good but rather to ask what each individual requires to flourish and honor that as I meet and interact with each new energy.*

7. After you are finished, blow out the candle. Feel confident that kaffir lime leaf, air, fire, Tara, and the animal archetype Red Dragonfly are indeed actively engaged in supporting you in your efforts to understand how to best be in service to humankind.

Invoking Fire Energy with a Candle Ritual

Fire can represent many things, such as bringing warmth to a situation, being passionate about something, or burning away something that no longer serves. In this fire ritual, the characteristics of the tools you use—the color of the candle, the type of essential oil, the number of drops, and the affirmations and incantations you use—help focus and direct the energy with which you would like to work.

Candle Ritual

1. Light an unscented candle. Allow the wax to puddle, then blow out the flame. Add to the wax whichever essential oil supports your intention. For example, you might use kaffir lime leaf to help you overcome a limiting behavior, agarwood for understanding emotional entanglement, galangal for playfulness, betel leaf for working with shadow, massoia bark for dream work, rose for working with the bright aspects of the divine feminine, vetiver for grounding, pink pepper seed for positive sexuality . . . the possibilities are many. The number of drops of essential oil that you add to the wax will be dictated by the vibration you're looking for (see pages 174–75).

2. Once you've added the drops of essential oil to the hot wax, focus on the aroma and the energy it brings. Depending on the energy you are invoking, you may wish to include mantras, affirmations, archetypal images, and so on.

Enlivening a Candle

As an extension of the candle ritual, you could carve tattva symbols into the side of the candle while repeating a mantra or affirmation, calling upon the overlying energy of the essential oil's archetype to enliven your candle. Thereafter, every time you light that candle, its energy will amplify the energy with which you are working. For example, say you are going through a difficult emotional time due to a thorny breakup.

You could choose a pink candle for your candle ritual because it promotes self-love. You could then carve a triangle within a circle on the side (air with the seed of fire, the sacred geometry of kaffir lime leaf) to cut any energetic cording that is keeping you bound to the other. Then carve a square with a crescent moon and circle inside (earth with the seed of water and air, the sacred geometry of massoia bark) to allow yourself to be dynamically reorganized to the most beneficial energetic arrangement. If you then use this enlivened candle in the candle ritual, adding the essential oils whose sacred geometry you have carved on the candle to the hot wax will amplify the practice.

Invoking a Meditative State with a Flame-Gazing Ritual

There are many reasons to meditate: coming clear on a nagging problem, understanding more deeply who you really are, clearing your mind, pondering spiritual mysteries, or merging with the divine. The possibilities are endless.

We use black or white candles here to invoke the energy of two powerful portals to your greatest wisdom: water and ether. As you will remember, water (white) is the soul and the collective unconscious, and ether (black) is spirit and akasha. The two suggested essential oils, frankincense and Chinese rice flower, offer powerful vibrations to support your journey into self and the universe.

Ingredients

Frankincense or Chinese rice flower essential oil

Flame Gazing

1. Light a white or black candle. Let the wax puddle, then add frankincense or Chinese rice flower essential oil. Which oil you choose and the number of drops you use will depend on your specific intent and the focus of your meditation. You might want to clear your

mind, ask what number would be of most benefit, and let it come to mind. Then look up the number to help set your intent for your meditation.

2. Gaze at the flame with unfocused eyes until your eyes tear up. Then close your eyes and allow your mind to "melt" into silence as if the noise had been burned away, enjoying the deep meditative state.

Quick Rituals for When You Are on the Go

Sometimes you don't have the time for a full meditative ritual. Other times you know that you face a consistent daily difficulty, like a trying commute, that you'd like to face with patience and calm. In these cases, these vibrational healing rituals can offer quick energetic support.

Quick-Hit Aromatherapy Ritual

This quick practice could be especially useful in situations where, for example, you use blue chamomile, which stimulates the throat chakra, to settle your nerves and find your voice before speaking in public. Or, for another example, if you know that you are about to have a difficult conversation, you could use massoia bark to amplify structured dynamism—this oil helps you respond in the moment so that you can quickly adapt to all the energy and information coming at you. Or if you are getting ready to garden, you may wish to amplify your ability to commune with nature by trying kaffir lime leaf.

1. If you are on the go and just need a little shot of energetic adjustment, you can simply uncap an appropriate bottle of essential oil and breathe in deeply, infusing yourself with the energy you would like to invoke.

2. Then, if possible, look upon the tattva symbol (in my commerical

line of essential oils for stimulating the tattvas, the sacred geometry is printed right on the bottle for this very purpose) for five seconds, and you are good to go!

Quick Invocation Ritual

This ritual for energizing or healing a space or item could not be more simple or flexible. You could use it, for example, with lavender in a bedroom to protect against nightmares, with black pepper in your office to promote success, or with sandalwood in your meditation area for profound revelation.

1. Apply one drop of the essential oil whose energy you wish to invoke to the palms of your hands. Rub your palms together, creating friction, until the scent is diffused.
2. Hold out your hands with the palms flat and facing up. Breathe in deeply, then repeat the mantra of that essential oil out loud over your palms. Repeat until your palms feel enlivened with the essential oil's energy.
3. When you feel ready, slowly and steadily move your hands over the area or item you wish to infuse with healing energy.

Keep in mind that all the rituals I've described in this chapter are only examples. There are endless combinations of tools, intentions, and practices. Also, feel free to layer methods. For example, you could use a candle ritual and a bathing ritual together, or personal anointing and flame gazing, to amplify the energy of any essential oil. I encourage you to experiment with the different base and essential oil combinations and the various ritual delivery methods. Experimentation helps awaken your inner alchemist!

Sample Practice:
Application of Knowledge

The following is a simple example of a practice built around betel leaf and its associated elements and how we can invoke its archetypal pattern to facilitate a change.

An individual comes to the awareness that she overidentifies with her body as an object to be admired for its appearance. She realizes that she has become increasingly stuck in and agitated by this energy as she has aged and her body has changed. This realization disturbs her in many ways, from its effect on her primary love relationship (her desire for physical intimacy has faded due to embarrassment about her appearance) to the way in which she interacts with others. Suddenly, she finds herself acutely aware of everyone else's age and physical appearance, and strong emotions such as jealousy and anger are surfacing in her. These unpleasant and confusing emotions are compounded by her lack of a strong sense of self and the knowledge of what makes her uniquely wonderful beyond her body. She realizes how much energy she has tied up in understanding self from that perspective, and she wants to shift it.

For this woman, one of the most difficult pieces of healing has already been accomplished: discovering the disharmonic pattern. (If she were still searching for the cause, betel leaf could support this process.)

She decides to start her healing process by addressing this issue where she feels it has the tightest grip: the distorted fire element (ego grasping) that makes her cling to her youth and resist the natural progression of self and the gifts that each stage brings. She concludes that this energy is rooted in the misidentification and misunderstanding of the body in relation to the overall understanding of self. After careful consideration, she decides to build her healing ritual using betel leaf essential oil as the focal point, supported by almond oil as the base oil, using personal anointing or aura misting as the delivery method. Because betel leaf holds the energy of fire and fire produces the ego, betel leaf can relieve fire-based maladies—in this example, the sense of how she relates to her physical body. Betel leaf will allow this woman to see herself with fresh eyes and appreciate her natural aging process. Almond base oil supports aging with grace and allows for this to be a joyful journey.

She creates a quiet, sacred space for blending the oils and for meditation. To enliven the essential oil blend as she prepares it, she first holds a clear glass bowl in her hands and visualizes her intent to clear away the disharmonic energies that pollute her well-being. Next, she pours one teaspoon of almond base oil into the bowl, while invoking the energy of almond: *Almond, help dissolve the bonds of fear of aging due to the changing form of my body; give me the grace to see the deeper beauty I possess, to be liberated from this destructive illusion, and to joyfully inhabit every moment and every stage of my life.* (Simply speak from the heart; this invocation is only an example.)

Next, she adds to the almond oil six drops of betel leaf essential oil. (The number six holds the vibration of reorganization of self.) As she deliberately counts out the drops, she deeply takes in betel leaf's scent and acknowledges its healing gifts: *Betel leaf, I have been abducted by my ego and caught in illusion and despair due to my aging body. My heart aches, and I cannot find solace, as I am preoccupied by my appearance, and it steals the joy from my life. With your strong medicine of shifting deeply rooted ways of being, please help liberate me from this ensnarement, that I might have the eyes to truly see all of who I am and see the beauty and joy in what I find.* (Again, simply speak from the heart; this invocation is only an example.)

She uses her the middle finger of her left hand to blend the energies of the almond and betel leaf oils, as the middle finger promotes stability within the self when you are undergoing changes and working to lift limiting beliefs.

When she is ready, she lights a white, unscented candle and adds three drops of betel leaf essential oil to the softened wax to further enhance the purification ritual. Sitting on a low cushion, she holds the bowl containing the essential oil mixture and repeats the betel leaf incantation aloud the three times, to further enliven the blend: *Dear betel leaf, please support me in honestly assessing all aspects of self, including ego-driven behaviors and the dark aspects of my personality. Help me to have the strength to find my weaknesses and to understand that the magic lies within this very act of honest self-introspection.*

This act of intense self-love—loving yourself enough to do difficult work because you know you are worth the gifts it will bring—leads the way to understanding, healing, and transmutation of shadow energy, allowing a new way of being to emerge. This is the Dark Goddess's path of awakening.

She then applies her blend to her wrists (for inhaling the aroma) and to the third chakra, at the solar plexus, in a counterclockwise motion. The third chakra is the place in the body where ego-born dysfunctions can be dynamically shifted, and as she applies the oil blend she focuses on this intention.

Next, she asks her chosen divine archetype for assistance, respectfully acknowledging the archetype's ability to help.

She then recites the sacred syllable of fire, *ram,* which calls forth radical form shift—the destruction of matter. When speaking this syllable, she visualizes breaking down deeply habituated causation patterns that operate on a subconscious level and being freed from the compulsive behavior that has abducted her free will.

She closes her eyes, deeply inhales the scent of the essential oil from her wrist, and speaks the syllable *ham,* the sacred syllable of ether, which resonates to the endless possibilities of reformatting the energetic self (this action is supported by the seed of ether in betel leaf). Changes in the energetic self will, in turn, dictate physical, emotional, and mental behavioral changes.

Finally, she smells the essential oil on her wrist again and visualizes the changes she clarified in the ether (dark moon) phase being birthed from abstract knowing into the concrete as new behaviors. She then sits in silence or meditation, absorbing her new way of being. She acknowledges the shift and thanks all of the energies involved.

❧

Every individual processes differently; therefore, the number of healing sessions required to shift aspects of the self will differ. The combination of elements with which you work, your personal body type (dosha), and how deeply ingrained a behavior is are all factors to consider. As you move forward, continually wearing the oil blend you've created or working with a mister of the essential oil(s) you've chosen is a wonderful way to support and keep active the energy with which you are working.

Resources

SUGGESTED HEALERS

Candice Covington: Chakra balancing and aromatherapy sessions, flower essence treatments, phone consultations, and ongoing education classes. *Email:* candice@divinearchetypes.com. *Website:* https://divinearchetypes.org.

Cathy Kinnaird: Human design charts and interpretation. *Website:* www.humandesignnw.com.

Chopra Center: Programs that address body, mind, and spirit with an emphasis on utilizing nature (essential oils, base oils, and herbs), meditation, and ayurveda in a retreat setting; also have a top-notch team of M.D.'s who combine these timeless healing modalities with Western medicine. *Website:* www.chopra.com.

Christine G. Glenn, Psy.D.: Jungian counseling and dream interpretation. *Website:* www.christineglennphd.com.

M. Kelley Hunter: Astrology, specializing in working with the Dark Goddess. *Website:* http://heliastar.com.

Rosemary Beam: Education and rejuvenation; Earth-based and shamanistic healing techniques. *Website:* http://rising-fire.com.

Susan Johnson: Intuitive counselor with vast knowledge and background working with my system and tools; she also has the rare gift of being a true intuitive and guide in the process of life. She offers phone sessions. *Email:* masuzaki@comcast.net.

SUGGESTED HEALING TOOLS

Divine Archetypes: Esoteric essential oils and flower essences lovingly and mindfully handcrafted for invoking archetypes, working with the tattvas, and stimulating your chakras, as discussed in this book. *Website:* https://divinearchetypes.org.

Honoring the Sacred: Jewelry from the heart, especially designed for healing and spiritual growth. *Website:* http://honoringthesacred.com.

Notes

Chapter 1. Spiritual Alchemy:
Transmuting Our Inner Matrix

1. Dictionary.com, s.v. "Alchemy." http://dictionary.reference.com/browse /alchemy (accessed July 19, 2017).
2. Chopra, *The Spontaneous Fulfillment of Desire*, 38.
3. Hamerman, "Musicality of Living Processes."
4. Whitmont, *The Symbolic Quest*, 246.
5. Sheldrake, *A New Science of Life*, 55.
6. Powers, *A Concise Introduction to Tibetan Buddhism*, 141.
7. Jung, *The Collected Works*, 79.
8. Sheldrake, "Part 1: Mind, Memory, and Archetype Morphic Resonance and the Collective Unconscious."
9. Cashford, *The Moon*, 358.
10. Cashford, *The Moon*, 101.
11. Cashford, *The Moon*, 354.
12. Spilsbury, *The Mayan Oracle*, 293.
13. Caddy, *Flight into Freedom and Beyond*, 11.
14. Jung, *Aion*, 261.

Chapter 2. Divine Archetypes:
Harnessing the Power of the Gods

1. Powers, *A Concise Introduction to Tibetan Buddhism*, 77.
2. Preece, *The Psychology of Buddhist Tantra*, 191–92.
3. Preece, *The Psychology of Buddhist Tantra*, 191.

4. George, *Mysteries of the Dark Moon,* 180.

5. George, *Mysteries of the Dark Moon,* 181.

Chapter 3. Tattvas: Connecting with the Five Great Elements

1. Franz, *Alchemy,* 65.

2. Tiwari, *Ayurveda,* 5.

3. Bush, "Sunset," from album *Aerial.*

4. Moby, "We Are All Made of Stars," from album *18.*

5. Crossman and Barou, *Tibetan Mandala,* 36.

6. Tiwari, *Ayurveda,* 9.

7. Satyasangananda, *Tattwa Shuddhi,* 56.

8. Satyasangananda and Satyananda, *Tattwa Shuddhi: The Tantic Practice of Inner Purification,* 67.

9. Chodron, *How to Free Your Mind,* 19.

10. Crossman and Barou, *Tibetan Mandala,* 12.

11. Crossman and Barou, *Tibetan Mandala,* 13–14.

12. Landaw and Weber, *Images of Enlightenment,* 42.

Chapter 5. Emptiness: Releasing Consciousness from Matter

1. Shore, "An Absurdist Pantomime," 158.

2. Talbot, *The Holographic Universe,* 287.

3. Talbot, *The Holographic Universe,* 54–55.

4. Talbot, *The Holographic Universe,* 55.

5. Rinchen, *The Heart Sutra,* 90–91.

6. Franz, *Alchemy,* 47.

7. Rinchen, *The Heart Sutra,* 25.

Chapter 6. Essential Oils for Spiritual Alchemy

1. Hemenway, *Hindu Gods,* 86.

2. George, *Mysteries of the Dark Moon,* 66–67.

3. Schnaubelt, *Advanced Aromatherapy,* 48–49.

4. Hageneder, *The Meaning of Trees,* 142.

5. Hageneder, *The Meaning of Trees,* 42.

Chapter 9. Self-Study: Identifying Your Tattvic Arrangement

1. Johari, *Breath, Mind, and Consciousness,* 32.

2. Johari, *Breath, Mind, and Consciousness,* 32.

Chapter 10. Deepening Connections: Working with the Tattvas

1. Satyasangananda, *Tattwa Shuddhi,* 28.

2. Frawley, *Yoga and Ayurveda,* 82–83.

Chapter 14. Mantras and Yantras: Amplification Practices

1. Frawley and Lad, *The Yoga of Herbs,* 95.

2. Frawley and Lad, *The Yoga of Herbs,* 96.

3. Frawley, *Ayurveda and the Mind,* 232–33.

4. Dewar, *Trainings in Compassion,* 69–70.

Chapter 17. Rituals: Crafting a Unique Practice with Essential Oils

1. Stewart, *Healing Oils of the Bible,* 33.

Bibliography

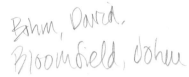

Bohm, David.
Bloomfield, John

Balz, Rodolphe. *The Healing Power of Essential Oils.* Twin Lakes, Wis.: Lotus Light, 1996.

Beck, Renee, and Sydney Barbara Metrick. *The Art of Ritual.* Berkeley, Calif.: Celestial Arts, 2003.

Bolen, Jean Shinoda. *Gods in Everyman: Archetypes That Shape Men's Lives.* New York: HarperCollins Publishers, 1989.

Bush, Kate "Sunset," *Ariel.* New York: Sony/ATV Music Publishing, 2005.

Caddy, Eileen. *Flight into Freedom and Beyond.* 2nd ed. Forres, Scotland: Findhorn Press, 2007.

Carroll, Lewis. *Alice's Adventures in Wonderland & Through the Looking-Glass.* New York: Signet Classics, 1960.

Cashford, Jules. *The Moon: Myth and Image.* New York: Four Walls Eight Windows, 2002.

Chodron, Thubten. *How to Free Your Mind: Tara the Liberator.* Ithaca, N.Y.: Snow Lion Publications, 2005.

Chopra, Deepak. *The Spontaneous Fulfillment of Desire: Harnessing the Infinite Power of Coincidence.* New York: Three Rivers Press, 2003.

Crossman, Sylvie, and Jean-Paul Barou, eds. *Tibetan Mandala: Art and Practice.* Translated by Rosetta Translations. Old Saybrook, Conn.: Konecky & Konecky, 2004.

Dewar, Tyler. *Trainings in Compassion: Manuals on the Meditation of Avalokiteshvara.* Ithaca, N.Y.: Snow Lion Publications, 2004.

Emoto, Masaru. *The Hidden Messages in Water.* Translated by David A. Thayne. Hillsboro, Ore.: Beyond Words Publishing, 2004.

Franz, Marie-Louise von. *Alchemy*. Toronto: Inner City Books, 1980.

Frawley, David. *Ayurveda and the Mind: The Healing of Consciousness*. Twin Lakes, Wis.: Lotus Press, 1996.

———. *Yoga and Ayurveda: Self-Healing and Self-Realization*. Twin Lakes, Wis.: Lotus Press, 1999.

Frawley, David, and Vasant Lad. *The Yoga of Herbs: An Ayurvedic Guide to Herbal Medicine*. 2nd ed. Twin Lakes, Wis.: Lotus Press, 1988.

George, Demetra. *Mysteries of the Dark Moon: The Healing Power of the Dark Goddess*. New York: HarperOne, 1992.

Guttman, Ariel, and Kenneth Johnson. *Mythic Astrology Applied: Personal Healing through the Planets*. St. Paul, Minn.: Llewellyn Publications, 2004.

Hageneder, Fred. *The Meaning of Trees: Botany. History. Healing. Lore*. San Francisco, Calif.: Chronicle Books, 2005.

Halevi, Z'ev Ben Shimon. *The School of Kabbalah*. Boston: Red Wheel/Weiser, 1986.

Hamerman, Warren J. "Musicality of Living Processes." *21st Century Science and Technology* 2, no. 2 (March–April 1989).

Hemenway, Priya. *Hindu Gods: The Spirit of the Divine*. San Francisco: Chronicle Books, 2003.

Johari, Harish. *Breath, Mind, and Consciousness*. Rochester, Vt.: Destiny Books, 1989.

Jung, Carl G. *The Collected Works*. Edited by Sir Herbert Read, Michael Fordham, and Gerhard Adler. Vol. 9, part 1, *The Archetypes and the Collective Unconscious*. Translated from the German by R. F. C. Hull. New York: Routledge, 2014. First published in England in 1959 by Routledge & Kegan Paul.

Jung, Carl G., Gerhard Adler, and R. F. C. Hull. *Aion: Researches into the Phenomenology of the Self*. 2nd ed. Princeton, N.J.: Princeton University Press, 1969.

Kaminski, Patricia. *Flowers That Heal: How to Use Flower Essences*. Dublin: Newleaf, 1998.

Landaw, Jonathan, and Andy Weber. *Images of Enlightenment: Tibetan Art in Practice*. Ithaca, N.Y.: Snow Lion Publications, 1993.

Moby. "We Are All Made of Stars," *18*. London: Mute, 2002.

Mumford, Jonn. *Magical Tattwas: A Complete System of Self-Development.* St. Paul, Minn.: Llewellyn Publications, 1997.

Powers, John. *A Concise Introduction to Tibetan Buddhism.* Ithaca, N.Y.: Snow Lion Publications, 2008.

Preece, Rob. *The Psychology of Buddhist Tantra.* Ithaca, N.Y.: Snow Lion Publications, 2006.

Rinchen, Sonam. *The Heart Sutra.* Edited and translated by Ruth Sonam. Ithaca, N.Y.: Snow Lion Publications, 2003.

Satyasangananda, Saraswati. *Tattwa Shuddhi.* Munger, Bihar, India: Yoga Publications Trust, 1984.

Satyasangananda, Saraswati, and Saraswati Satyananda. *Tattwa Shuddhi: The Tantric Practice of Inner Purification.* Munger, Bihar, India: Yoga Publications Trust, 2003.

Schnaubelt, Kurt. *Advanced Aromatherapy.* Rochester, Vt.: Healing Arts Press, 1998.

Sheldrake, Rupert. *A New Science of Life: The Hypothesis of Formative Causation.* Los Angeles: J. P. Tarcher, 1981.

———. "Part 1: Mind, Memory, and Archetype Morphic Resonance and the Collective Unconscious." *Psychological Perspectives* 18, no. 1 (Spring 1987): 9–25. www.sheldrake.org/research/morphic-resonance/part-i-mind-memory -and-archetype-morphic-resonance-and-the-collective-unconscious (accessed July 20, 2017).

Shore, Barbara. "An Absurdist Pantomime: The Collision of Violence, Innocence, and Pseudoinnocence." In *Psychology at the Threshold.* Edited by Dennis Patrick Slattery and Lionel Corbett. Carpinteria, Calif.: Pacifica Graduate Institute Publications, 2010.

Slattery, Dennis Patrick, and Lionel Corbett, eds. *Psychology at the Threshold.* Carpinteria, Calif.: Pacifica Graduate Institute Publications, 2010.

Spilsbury, Ariel. *The Mayan Oracle.* Santa Fe, N.Mex.: Bear & Company, 1992.

Stewart, David. *Healing Oils of the Bible.* Marble Hill, Mo.: Care Publications, 2002.

Talbot, Michael. *The Holographic Universe.* New York: HarperPerennial, 1992.

Tierra, Michael. *Planetary Herbology.* Edited by David Frawley. Twin Lakes, Wis.: Lotus Press, 1988.

Tiwari, Maya. *Ayurveda: A Life of Balance*. Rochester, Vt.: Healing Arts Press, 1995.

Whitmont, Edward C. *The Symbolic Quest: Basic Concepts of Analytical Psychology*. New York: Putnam for the C. G. Jung Foundation for Analytical Psychology, 1969.

Worwood, Valerie Ann. *The Fragrant Mind: Aromatherapy for Personality, Mind, Mood, and Emotion*. Novato, Calif.: New World Library, 1996.

Index